The Weight Is Over

An *Eating Energy!* Approach to Fat-Loss and Optimal Health Featuring the FitTest™

Dr. Jack Tips, CCN

For information address:

Apple-A-Day Press
3654 Bee Caves Road, Suite D
Austin, Texas 78746-5371

ISBN 0-929167-19-8

Library of Congress Cataloging-in-Publication Data

Tips, Jack C.
The Weight Is Over; non fiction, self help / Jack Tips
p. cm.
ISBN 0-929167-19-8
1. Diet — health aspects 2. Diet — physiological aspects 3. Diet Therapy — physiological aspects 4. Food — health aspects 5. Nutrition — health aspects 6. Nutritionally-induced diseases
I. Title

99-095493

First Edition

Editor: Cathy Buettner, Say It Well, Austin, Texas
Typesetting, Lay Out: Keith Bahlmann, Bahl Graphics, Austin, Texas
Proofreading: Janine Tips / Sashi Kimball, Austin, Texas
Jacket Design: Dwayne and Stephanie Roecker, Graphic Edge, Inc., Austin, Texas
Printer: Print Haus Inc., Austin, Texas

This information is provided in good will for informational and educational purposes only.

ACKNOWLEDGEMENTS

I thank **God** for life and the perfect order of the Natural Laws of Life that govern our health. Knowing there is a perfect plan, chaos included, means that we can exercise our free will and know the truth. There are clear answers to nutritional confusion and, in this gift of life, we can experience our very best expression of vitality and health. Also, special thanks to my loving parents, Craig and Ruth Ann and my brother William for their loving support.

My wife, **Janine**, gave me the time, space, and support necessary to write. She is my haven and her love is my muse. This book was written while moving our residence. Can you believe the depths of her heart and devotion? Thank you. I love you.

Thanks to three very special men, **Todd Stanwood, Lou DeCaprio, and Scott Stanwood**, the founders of Ideal Health International, Inc., who allowed me to communicate part of their dream to improve the health of the world, one test at a time.

Thanks to **Dr. Alexander Bralley**, one of the world's great nutritional biochemists, for bringing forth the FitTest© and helping empower individuals with nutritional knowledge and self-destiny in improving their health.

Special thanks to fellow nutritionist **Denise Autry, RN, CCN**, for being a second opinion.

Thanks to **Sashi Kimball**, who read the rough draft and gave her two-cents'-worth of valuable advice.

My heartfelt gratitude and deepest appreciation is hereby expressed to **Dr. Stuart Wheelwright**, a mentor now departed, most deeply respected, who, with his provocative and iconoclastic insights, ignited the spark that launched my fifteen-year quest for understanding the role of nutrition in optimal health.

Finally, a thanks of admiration to my editor, **Cathy Buettner**, who took on this project under difficult circumstances and gave it her all. More than just editing my ramblings, she put her heart into this project and made it something special.

DEDICATIONS

This book is dedicated to my beautiful wife Janine, my cherished companion whom I dearly love;

also to my daughter Lauren – the equestrian;

my stepson, Ryan – the guitarist;

my stepdaughter, Jessica – the retired gymnast turned teenager;

and my son Colin - no longer present but my love knows no bounds.

Each of you is a light in the window of my life.

This book is also dedicated to all people who seek to improve their health and have the insight to know that nutrition is fundamental to the quality of life.

And for you? May this book be a blessing in your life.

CONTENTS

PART ONE
Rev Up Your Fat Burning Machine

CHAPTER EIGHT

Protein's Role in Fat Burning and Health 139

CHAPTER NINE

Protein: Health and Fat Loss Tips 157

CHAPTER TEN

Fats' Fabulous Role in Fat-Burning 163

Part One

Rev Up Your Fat Burning Machine

INTRODUCTION

The Weight Is Over

Truth is the property of no individual but is the treasure of all. - R.W. Emerson

Now You Can Lose Weight While You Sleep!

Does this sound like a dream come true; or does it sound too good to be true? Does this sound like another sensationalized magazine story? Sure it does, but consider this. What if it's true?

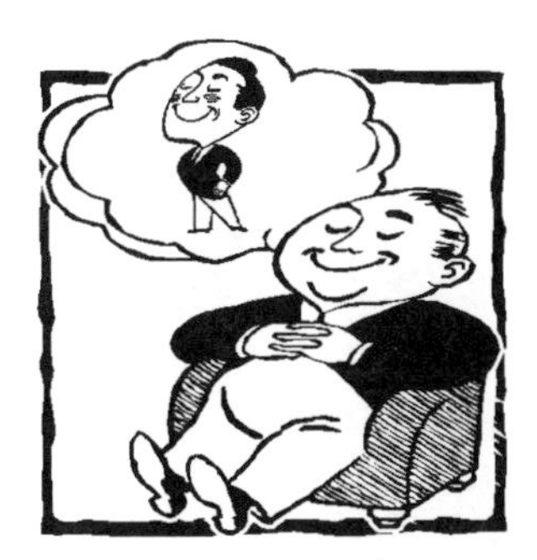

Actually, it is true! Breakthroughs in nutritional science conclusively show how you can regain your body's ability to burn stored fat and unleash the energy within your cells for optimal health. It's simple! It's easy! In *The Weight Is Over* you'll learn how to win the health-freedom you deserve.

It doesn't involve eating fat-free foods or counting calories. It doesn't involve high impact aerobics or jogging for miles, and it doesn't involve starving! It does involve a 10 inch disk and what proportions you put on it.

You guessed it – the 10-inch disk is your plate and how much of what foods go on it.

Now I know that you're hoping to hear that you must divide your plate into three equal portions – ice cream, pizza, and chips, but let's be realistic. To ensure you'll take a look at this plan and see how simple and delicious it is, I'll give you this preview (my humble opinion) - you'll love it; you'll love the results; **and** you'll get back some of the foods you've been mistakenly told are bad for you! Sounds interesting, doesn't it? Keep reading and you'll see how this plan can work for you.

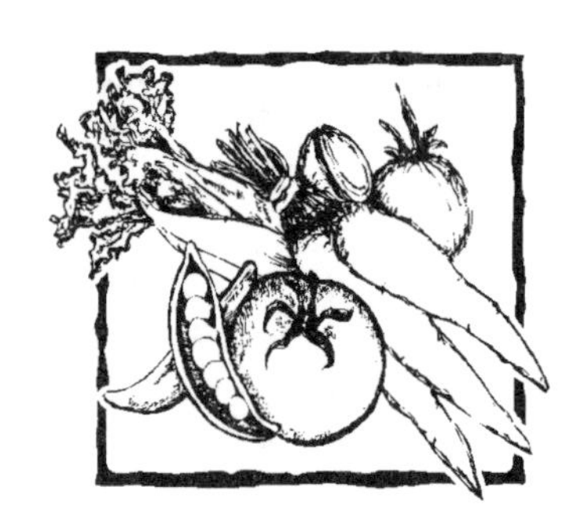

This book is but one part of a larger work, *Eating Energy*, a book that shows you how to redesign your health from the ground up. In *The Weight Is Over*, we'll focus on an immediate problem and an immediate solution with the urgency and results you need! In *The Weight Is Over*, you can start losing weight and increasing your energy, now. You can continue learning in more detail how nutrition holds the answers to health, vitality, and longevity from *Eating Energy*, if you're interested.

The side effect of proper nutrition is proper burning of fat! The side effect of The Weight Is Over Program is the proper, increased burning of excess fat.

Can you really lose weight while you sleep? Absolutely! Your body burns 75% of its calories during sleep. All you have to do is *allow* your body to burn fat while you sleep (and while you're awake, too). The secret to accomplishing this dream is right at your fingertips. It's in the ratios of food you eat: the ratios of the three macro-nutrients – protein, fat, and carbohydrate.

The big question is: "What are the right ratios for you?" How do you find the magic balance that will unlock your fat-burning mechanism when your metabolism is unique? In the first few chapters, you'll learn how to determine in which ballpark your unique metabolism is playing. Once you're in the game, you can hit the nutritional homerun – lose weight while simultaneously building your health.

Frankly, there's a lot more at stake here than losing weight. Proper weight loss also improves health, not only due to less work for the heart, but because proper loss of excess fat improves all the metabolic processes and function of body systems, including the immune system. Proper weight loss is really fat loss, and fat loss is a side-effect of improving health through nutrition!

How to burn fat? You must eat your way out!

Right now, if you have too much fat-weight, chances are the way you are eating is pushing your nutrition into the fat-storage vault around your middle. Your body wants to access that fat for energy, but the vault is locked. Why is it locked? It's locked because your current eating habits activate the hormone that stores fat and keeps it stored, instead of activating the hormone that burns fat. Every meal is your choice. *The Weight Is Over* will teach you to make the choices that will unlock that fat storage vault and burn your unwanted and unnecessary fat stores.

Can you get a hormone shot? Nope. It's doesn't work that way because of the body's check-and-balance systems. The answer to who wins the heavyweight fight between Fat Storage vs. Fat Burning is found on your plate. Food is the most powerful modulator of the hormones that control fat. Therefore, you must eat your way out of having too much fat-weight! *The Weight Is Over* will show you how foods are a powerful ally in fat loss.

This book offers something *new!* Basically, everything I've said up to this point has been said before, but here is a nutritional breakthrough that, with scientific precision, makes it easier than ever before to lose fat-weight and optimize health. Now there is an affordable laboratory test that can score the key factors in your current fat-storage/fat-burner hormonal balance. From this score, you can custom-design your nutrition to accommodate fat burning instead of fat storage.

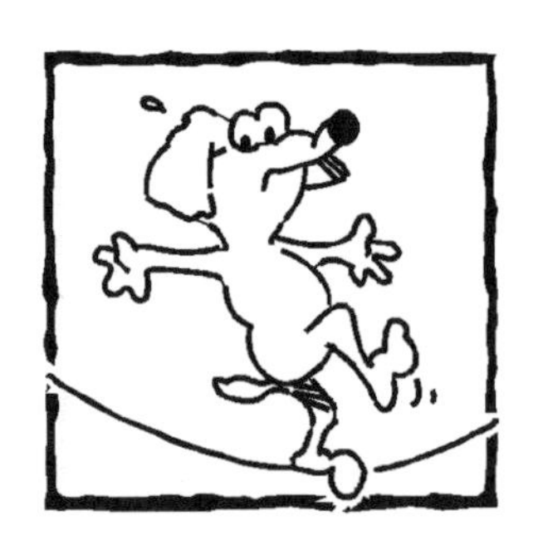

Weight loss has never been easier! You have never been so free to control your own destiny! If you have been trying to reduce fat in your diet with fat-free products and if you have been eating more pasta and potatoes to avoid foods with cholesterol, you have unwittingly been tipping your hormonal balance into the fat-storage mode! Sorry. Your good intentions have led you astray.

You see, one of the secrets to good nutrition is *balance*. We all need a balanced diet. That balance is not found in the basic Food Pyramid, the guiding force behind the diets that have caused Americans to gain an average of 10 pounds each over the past 12 years. The Food Pyramid is bottom heavy, just like people who eat that way.

Balance is an individual matter! A "one-size-fits-all" weight loss plan will leave many people (around 70%) floundering outside the ballpark gates. They don't even get in to see the game, much less play. A custom-designed, fat-burning plan is your entry ticket to the right ballpark where your hormones will load the bases and hit the nutritional home run for you.

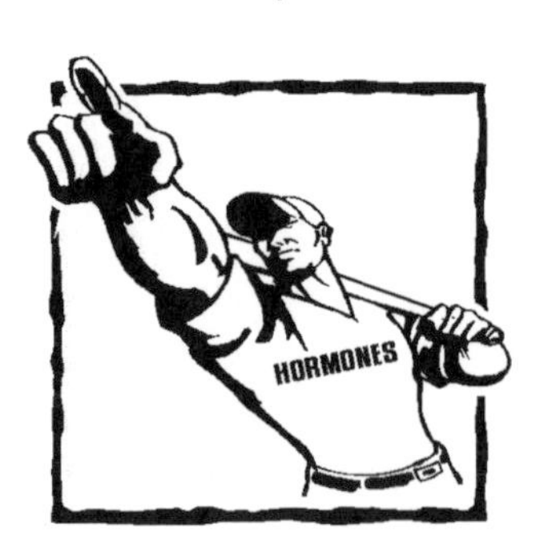

Eating to burn fat is really simple. It's not so much *what you eat*, but the *ratios of what you eat* that evoke your powerful hormonal response to either store or burn fat. As a nutritionist, I cringe when I emphasize that point, true as it may be, because I know that *what* you eat and the *quality* of what you eat is critically important to overall health. People making horrible food choices can still lose weight, but they won't build health. The fat-burning law works impartially — but here is your chance to optimize

It's not what you eat, but the balance or ratios *of what you eat that unleashes your powerful fat-burning mechanism. True, but...*

your weight and your health at the same time.

That statement about the proper ratio stresses only one of twelve dietary principles necessary for optimal health. It focuses on only one of twelve "spinning plates" that make up our "balancing act" of nutrition. On the other hand, the statement that *the ratios of what you eat control your fat burning* is exactly right. It is simply the *ratio* of macro-nutrients that holds the key to fat metabolism. Losing fat, for many people, can be as easy as reorganizing your plate.

Even though I'm bursting to share more information with you than you'll ever need, I'll keep our focus, as much as I can be restrained, on weight loss – fast, simple, easy, permanent! This is the condensed, quick-results information that can launch you on a nutritional adventure to improve how you look and feel, and how *long* you'll look and feel great!

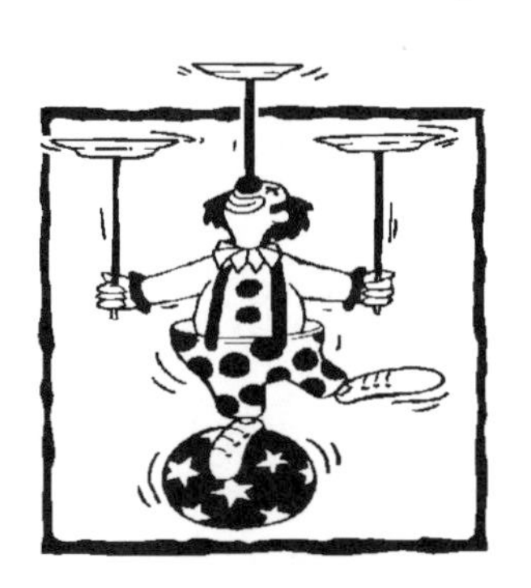

Your decision to read this book could be one of the most important choices in your life! This simple, first step can unleash a powerful ally to help you in your desire to have optimal weight and energy. Congratulations! I'm excited about sharing these vital principles on how you can create a new level of health and inner vitality that will enhance every moment of your life. Let's get started now!

About This Book . . .

You'll love this book if you:

- want to lose fat

- have failed previously with diets and want to know why most diets fail
- want science to validate your nutrition plan
- are tired of "experts" telling you what not to eat
- want freedom from chronic, degenerative diseases
- want to enjoy a more fulfilling life
- want to lose weight while sleeping
- need more energy
- appreciate results
- wonder why Americans eating the low-fat, high carbohydrate "healthy heart" diet are fatter than ever before in our history.

The purpose of the above list is to help you focus on your goals and appreciate that over 30 years of experience and research have gone into the information presented *in The Weight Is Over.* This is the tip of the iceberg, the crown; but the nutritional foundation for this plan is massive, as described in *Eating Energy.*

How This Book Is Structured

Part 1 presents the principles of fat-loss metabolism, shows you how to obtain a laboratory test that marks glucose metabolism, and prepares you to use the results to design the ratios of macronutrients (proteins/fats/carbohydrates) in your diet for optimal weight – a big step toward optimal health.

Part 2 presents detailed knowledge about the macro-nutrients so you can become an expert in choosing the foods that support your health.

Part 3 presents key insights on factors other than macro-nutrients that bring success in fat-reduction and in improving health.

It will help you tailor your diet to your specific goals, as well as build a custom-designed program to accelerate your results to lose fat and build health.

A Nutritional Solution to Health Concerns

Problems occur when a force disrupts the body's ability to keep all the metabolic plates spinning. Crash! A plate shatters on the floor. Symptoms such as weight gain, fatigue, gas, bloating, headaches, mood swings, and skin eruptions can occur, and, if prolonged, chronic degenerative diseases manifest, such as arthritis, diabetes, osteoporosis, arteriosclerosis and cancer.

What are the forces that disrupt our nutritional health balance? They are legion. Deficiencies or excesses in micro-nutrients (vitamins, minerals, trace minerals, enzymes, co-enzymes), water, oxygen, electromagnetic properties, or fiber, as well as imbalances in macro-nutrients (protein, carbohydrate, and fat) can quickly disrupt the spin of health.

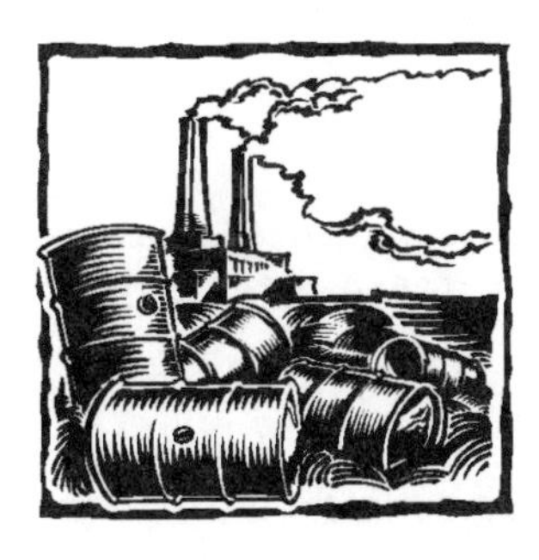

Other factors can also tax our detoxification processes and innate balance. These include stress, emotional upheaval and lifestyle issues such as smoking, excessive alcohol use and xenobiotic substances (preservatives, aspartame, food colorings, pesticides, drugs (prescription, recreational and over-the-counter), chemicals and non-nutritive additives, as well as heavy metals such as mercury, lead and aluminum.

Other causes of stress to our detoxification mechanisms include air pollution, radiation pollution, water pollution and chemical additives, and disruptive electromagnetic fields from power transformers. Whew! That's quite a list.

If we go even deeper, genetics and metabolic patterns also play a role in the spin of health. Thoughts, especially negative thoughts (such as anger, prolonged grief, jealousy, greed, resentment and self-pity) can all upset the expression of health, by altering metabolic processes.

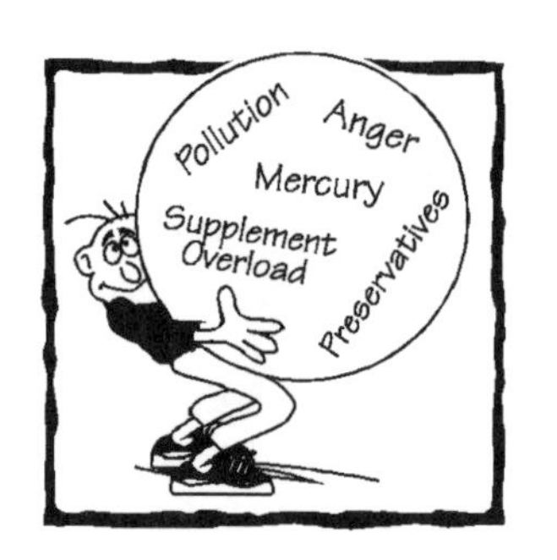

The job of the clinical nutritionist is to figure out which plate, or plates, are wobbling or have fallen, and, like the brilliant vaudeville performer, intervene with a corrective nutritional adjustment (therapy). The diagnostic method of the clinical nutritionist is laboratory testing. The remedy is found in food, nutritional supplements and natural therapies.

It is from this perspective that I will address the issues of fat loss and optimal nutrition simultaneously. Why this *simultaneous* distinction? Because the "pop nutrition" featured in many magazines and tabloids is lacking in true nutritional insight. "Pop nutrition" often gives us weight loss at the expense of health; it teaches us how to manipulate our bodies without significantly building vitality. The end result is an actual loss of our most precious state of being – our health.

It is time for the full story and, with it, the power to make both *weight (fat) corrections* and *health and vitality enhancements* at the same time. We must consider all the possibilities – to know the truth and then apply those simple, self-evident principles which so many seem to have overlooked.

This book will provide a plan to help you master proper nutrition so you can live a full and vital life. To do this, you'll need to understand the spinning plates of nutritional balance because times have changed and our society and lifestyles present a few obstacles to overcome. For simplicity's sake, let your body orchestrate the spin of the plates. Your job is to make sure that your body has the proper tools in the proper balance to do what it does best!

Despite the fact that we seem to live in a "sound bite" society which can operate on *fragments* of information, we really must have the *whole picture* for truly effective nutrition. A little knowledge is a dangerous thing. A solid understanding of the simple basics of nutrition is the power to live a healthy life. The nutritional insights of this book are not really astounding. They are just common sense. They are simple, but they bring freedom.

My proposal is this: Why don't we base our nutrition on scientific knowledge tempered with common sense, or ancient wisdom? If we desire to change our weight, let's base it on a laboratory test that can factually steer us to the most effective 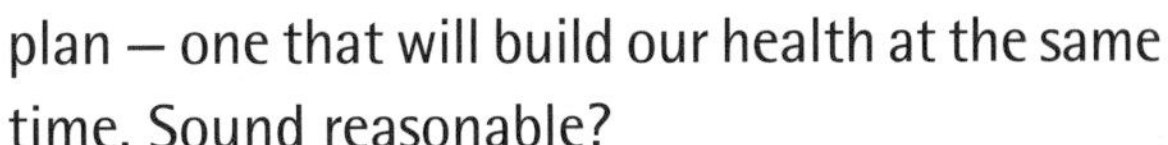 plan – one that will build our health at the same time. Sound reasonable?

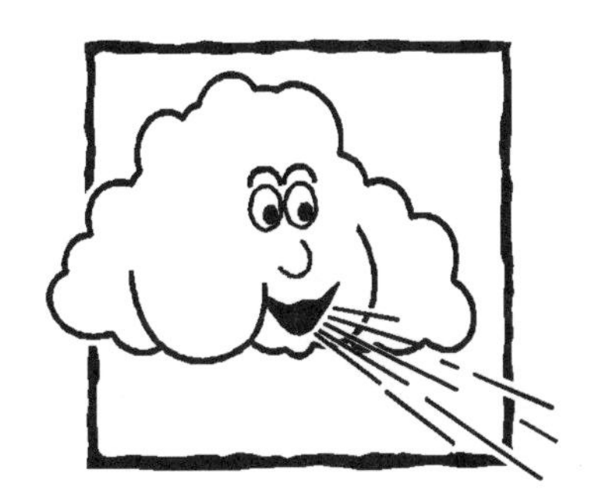

Great! So, hold on to your nutritional hat. The wind of change is about to blow and sweep us along into a wonderful world of delicious foods that promote a life of optimal weight, energy, mental clarity, longevity, and inherent joy. Since weight is such a big issue for so many people, we'll learn a shortcut to weight loss that doesn't sacrifice our health or short-change us in the long run.

Twelve years ago, I authored a 380-page nutritional book called *The Pro-Vita! Plan For Optimal Nutrition.* The book became a text for several natural health schools and earned the respect of a dedicated group of advocates who have experienced improved health and the remission of symptoms and disease as a result of its principles. It is now considered a nutrition classic (sounds like I'm ancient!). However, there's a good chance you've never heard of *The Pro-Vita! Plan For Optimal Nutrition.* From this, I learned a valuable lesson – one you'll appreciate. I've learned not to belabor the metabolic pathways and details that fascinate nutritionists, but bore the heck out of everyone else. My pledge to you is that this book will simplify lengthy nutritional issues, but refrain from oversimplifications.

Regarding Diet: It's what you do 80% of the time that sets the standard of your health.

Here's one simple nutritional insight that will help us avoid rigidity and often earns a sigh of relief. I'm happy to report that the reality of nutrition is this: it's what we do most, not all, of the time that sets our nutrition-standard. So let's establish a high quality standard! With an occasional indiscretion and an occasional "super food" thrown in, it all comes out in the wash. Our bodies are resilient. We have fabulous systems in place to maintain homeostasis (metabolic balance.) Let's focus on the genuinely important issues and let our bodies take care of the rest.

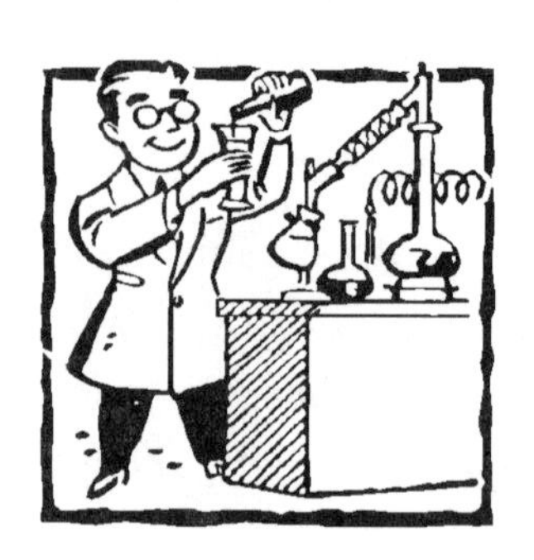

In Part One of this book you'll discover how to learn, via laboratory testing, what food plan will bring forth your optimal weight. More importantly, by applying true nutritional principles, the same food plan will build your optimal nutritional health, simultaneously! You *can* have it all – optimal weight, optimal health, all with the same simple plan!

So jump in! Today, you can take the most important steps in custom-designing your fat-loss/weight-optimizing nutritional plan.

Start Right Now!

In just a few minutes of reading, you'll have enough information to make a decision to take the FitTest and embark on a course of action that will nutritionally sculpt the best body you can have, as well as the most optimal dietary health you can experience. This is absolutely exciting!

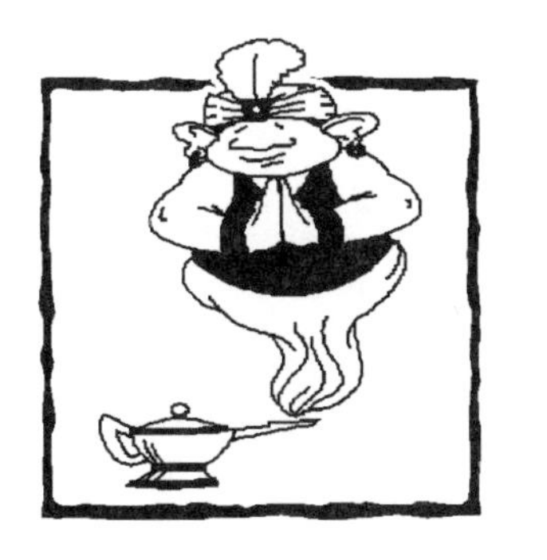

When you are ready, phone the toll-free number in The FitTest Chapter and get your lab kit on its way to you. Then begin applying the nutritional principles in the subsequent chapters. It won't be long before you experience how your body can thrive on sound nutrition.

Enjoy unleashing your health within! Come along now on a dietary sojourn that can change your life for the best of health. I am thrilled to be of service.

– *Jack Tips*

CHAPTER ONE

Spinning Plates

Try? There is no try.
There is only do, or do not. - Yoda

The Wheels Within Wheels Clockwork of Nutrition

Picture an outdoor vaudeville act. The performer spins fine china plates on skinny sticks. He stands a stick on the stage in front of him and spins the plate on its point. Miraculously, the stick remains upright and the plate doesn't fall. It stays spinning like a top in mid air. Then he does it again and again. More sticks and spinning plates line up. Soon, there are eight plates spinning. As long as the plates spin, they stay perched precariously on the sticks.

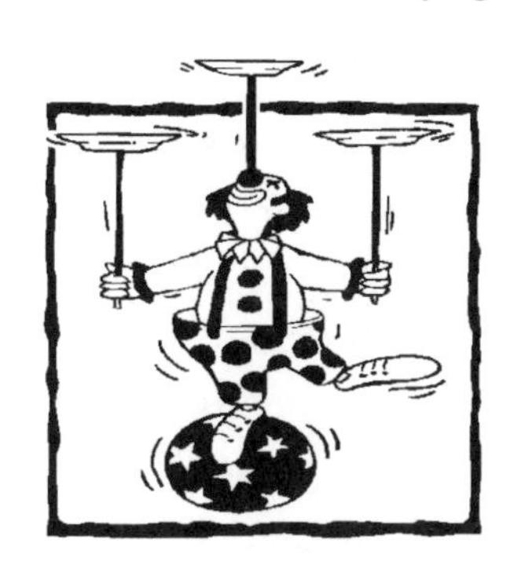

He refreshes the spin on the first plates and then starts another plate spinning and balances it on his forehead. Quickly he starts another and balances it on his foot. Two more are added, one in each hand. For one glorious minute, he is orchestrating 12 spinning plates. The music crescendos. The audience applauds.

Suddenly, a gust of wind blows across the stage. The performer deftly saves the act by adjusting the plates to account for the wind. The audience cheers. A train speeds by behind the stage. The stage shakes. But before the plates can fall off the sticks, the performer acrobatically adjusts and the plates remain upright, spinning, despite the tremor. The audience, already on their feet, realizes that not even the stage shaking can keep the masterful acrobat from a flawless performance. They not only applaud; they throw money and shout "Bravo!" in recognition of true mastery of an art.

Just think of all the physical laws operative in that moment of showmanship! The plates spin on sticks against the restriction of friction. Centrifugal force and centripetal force become a gyroscopic force. A breeze blows. Gravity pulls. The ground moves. The earth spins on its axis and circumnavigates the sun while the galaxy arcs its way through the spiral of time. So much to consider!

Human nutrition — a performance of spinning plates. No wonder confusion is the rule and so many diets bite the dust!

Such is human nutrition — a performance of spinning plates amid other rhythms and disruptive forces. Wheels within wheels of interdependent clockwork perform their vital functions amongst the ebb and flow of circadian rhythms and circulation of meridian energies. Plus, there are unexpected challenges to our nutritional state to which we must adapt. The nutrition plates spin simultaneously, and their various "nutrients" — protein, carbohydrates, fats, water, enzymes, fiber, hormones and other nutrients, air, vitamins, minerals, coenzymes, and electromagnetic energy — all perform their activities. Each spinning plate affects the others. No wonder nutrition is a confusing, contradictory tilt-a-whirl of information and opinions.

Further, the science of human nutrition is a frontier with the great unknown just beyond the border. Nutritional knowledge has doubled in the past fourteen months bringing forth many breakthroughs, but there are still many more questions than answers. The new research proves old ideas to be wrong and then, suddenly, proves some old, discarded ideas to be right after all.

The new nutritional discoveries keep marching our awareness toward the irrefutable fact that what we eat has a profound effect on our health, our emotions, and longevity. Nutrition is a high-stakes game: we can gain health-riches or we can suffer chronic degenerative diseases. What we do must be based on more certainty than a roll of the dice.

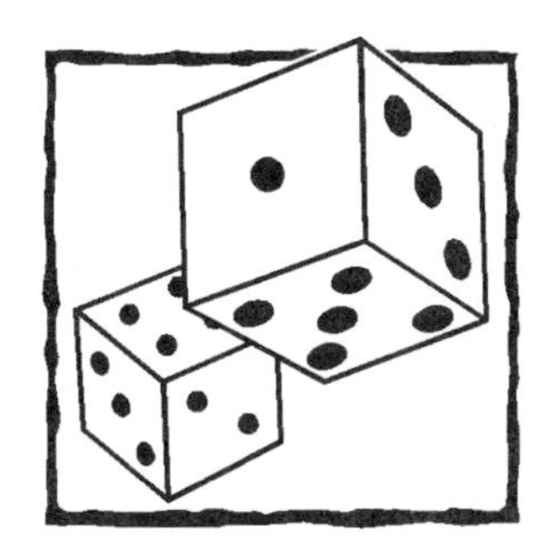

Into this budding science comes the usual over-exuberance of partial findings and misapplications of facts, as well as the uniquely human shortcoming of the belief that what works for one person works for another. This is where so many people have run into trouble, failure, and frustration in trying to apply the latest nutrition theory or fad. Practically any diet can work for 30% of the people. But that's not good enough, unless you're one of the 30%!

Nutrition and fat-loss follow exacting rules. When the diet is right, the fat will depart.

Your Body's Inherent Solution

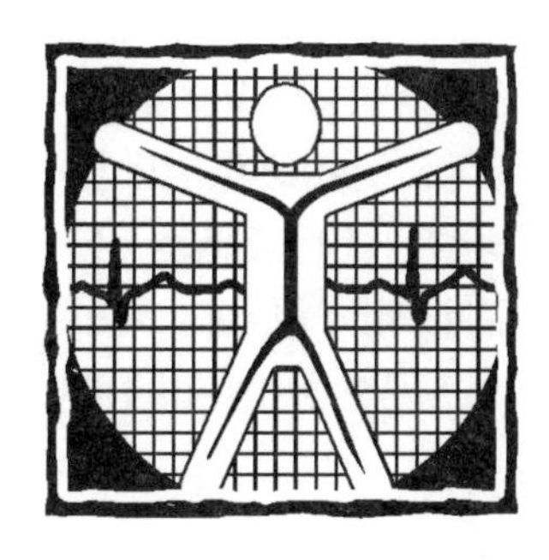

Despite the intricacies and complexities apparent in nutrition, and quite independent of our understanding or lack of it, our bodies have an inherent blueprint for maintaining the best of health. Even though we do not have all the pieces or fully understand the blueprint, our bodies already know how to keep all the plates spinning perfectly, provided there is not a disruptive force that throws things off balance. Thus, we must rely on the saving grace (self-preservation mechanism) of the body's inherent wisdom.

Given the right foods at the right time, our bodies are wizards at producing the best of health. This is the inherent blueprint at work. This is why nutrition is so important. What and how we eat predisposes our health significantly, barring a congenital defect or acquired disease as a sole cause of a symptom. When, despite the right foods, a person develops a disease, then medical, naturopathic, or homeopathic expertise is required.

Inherent within each of us is a self-regulating mechanism whose job is to adapt and maintain the best of health.

Just what is this inherent, innate, internal balancing principle? It has been identified by several names. *Homeostasis, equilibrium, vitality, vital force, self-preservation mechanism, balance, instinct,* and *it'll all come out in the wash* are a few of the scientific and not-so-scientific terms used to describe the body's ability to spin all the plates into a phenomenal state of well-being, and keep them spinning despite minor indiscretions.

The point here is that a human being should be able to live from day to day without being overly preoccupied with how to eat. Where in Nature does a polar bear go about the day wondering, "Am I eating too much fat?" When does a gnu ponder, "I wonder how many calories this tall grass has?" or a lion consider, "How many protein blocks can I eat with this gazelle?" or a shark say, "Let me consult my diet tables to see if I can eat fish on Monday."

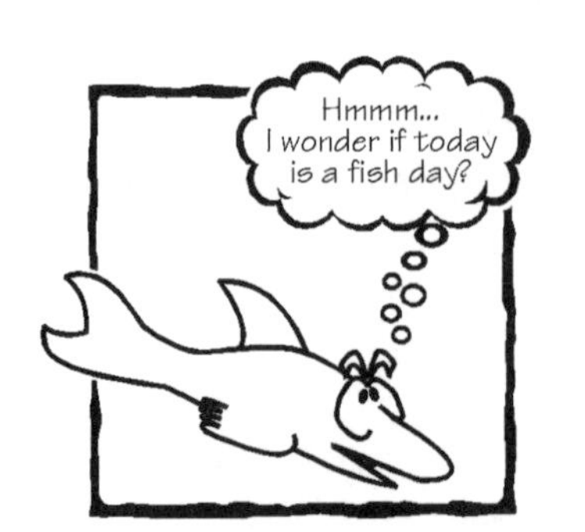

Why are human beings different? We're different because, in exercising our self-destiny, we've created some serious challenges that alter the spin of our health. However, instead of going back to the basics, many people erroneously believe that we can "crash diet" our way back to a better weight and more-optimal health without really changing the causes that brought the undesired results. We expect to play a beautiful song on a piano that's grossly out of tune by perfecting our technique, instead of tuning the piano first. Further, in trying to understand why our health is suffering, people often try to apply new, unproven technologies to bring a quick fix, rather than going back to the simple basics and letting their bodies fix the problem.

No one knows better than your body how to reduce fat and improve your health. Therefore, the key to unleashing your health within is to provide your body the tools so it can do its job. It really comes down to two things: remove the obstacles and provide the right tools – then the body can take care of itself.

Your body already knows how to open the door to access fat for energy and lose weight. Why is your foot against the door?

If only we can understand where and how we got off track, then we can correct the cause of the problem. Many people mistakenly think that they have several unrelated problems (for example: headaches, excessive fat around the middle, menstrual pain, aching joints, and elevated cholesterol.) When we go deeper into causes, it is not uncommon that all symptoms have a common cause – the body's inability to maintain health any better than its current state of health.

From this perspective, there are three factors that must spin properly for the body to correct its symptoms and restore optimal health.

- First, the foundational diet must be correct. Foods must provide all the *Eating Energy 12 Optimal Nutrition Factors*©. (Details later in this chapter.)

- Second, weak tissues must be identified, supported and repaired. This is accomplished with nutritional therapy.
- Third, the body's self-regulatory or healing mechanism must be focused to correct the cause of disturbance, to end its confusion, with the proper constitutional remedy. This is what the natural health movement is dedicated to – the healing of the whole person.

From this insightful overview comes *The Weight Is Over's* pathway to optimal fat loss that results in optimal weight and improved health.

Our focus in *The Weight Is Over* is to understand that fat gain or obesity is most often the body's perfect expression to the stimuli provided. The computer aphorism, "garbage in, garbage out" is applicable here. When we understand that fat-gain follows Natural Laws, we can alter the course of that process by applying the fat-burning Natural Laws. Rather than a see-saw approach of "Hormone Wars," let's set the stage for balance, then the body will deliver what we really want – **both** *optimal health* **and** *optimal weight.*

ShiftRight With The Eating Energy 12 Optimal Nutrition Factors©

One secret to making major improvements to your overall diet is to make small but valuable changes. These little changes need to be in crucial areas so the leverage you gain in improving your overall nutritional status is huge.

Everything that goes in your mouth can be viewed on a continuum, from left to right, arranged to show how detrimental or how beneficial that substance is to your nutritional health. For example, something commonly known to be detrimental for many people is a caffeinated soft drink. The sugar, caffeine, chemicals, artificial ingredients and lack of nutrients bring a stress to the body. On the other side, something beneficial for many people is a fresh garden salad. In this example, the soft drink falls on the left side with detrimental foods, and the salad falls on the right with the beneficial foods. For this analogy, if you wanted to improve your nutrition, you simply skip the soda and have some salad. This is a shift to the right, and the net gain in nutrition can be significant In fact, it can become the dividing line between health and disease.

I use the term "ShiftRight". What this means is that we rate all foods on a "health scale" and arrange them from left to right. Those on the left are the most detrimental. Those on the right are most beneficial. Here's the secret. To make a simple move toward better nutrition and health, all we have to do is delete a an item on the left side, add an item on the right, and the entire balance of the diet *shifts right* into a more optimal position.

This means that you don't have to make hundreds of changes all at once. All you have to do to *ShiftRight* is to gradually introduce beneficial foods while deleting a few detrimental foods. It also means that, often, the detrimental foods we crave can be gradually transitioned to the right to drop away when we're ready. When you ShiftRight into a more optimal nutritional lifestyle, you are rewarded with better energy and often, alleviation of symptoms. Here is a graphic example:

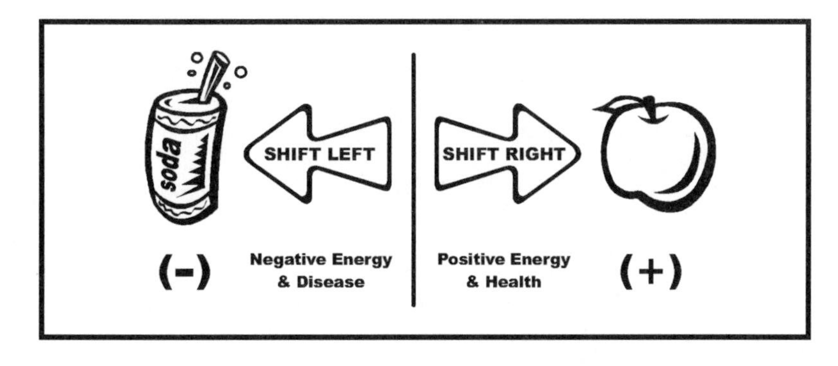

If a person deleted the caffeinated, sugar soda and ate an apple, the net gain nutritionally is a giant step in the ShifRight direction. If this were done over the course of a month, the net gain would be tremendous. Over the course of a year, the difference is phenomenal. You can see how the "center" of a person's diet can ShiftRight into the "Positive Energy & Health" dimension where healing best occurs.

The big question is this. How do we rate the foods? There are many factors that have a bearing on nutrition and the viability of a food to support health. We need some criteria for defining an overview of the complexities of nutrition in order to make it simple. What you are about to read is based on 30 years of my studies and quest to help people improve their health nutritionally. It provides the opportunity to understand the full nutritional picture as has never been done before. It is the basis of the ShiftRight Philosophy© that has helped thousands improve their health. It is called, "The *Eating Energy* 12 Optimal Nutrition Factors." I would like to share them with you now.

ShiftRight – delete a detrimental item on the left, add a beneficial item on the right. The entire dietary balance shifts right into a more optimal nutritional level.

The following scale can be used to assess a single food, an entire category of food, a meal – as well as an entire diet. Here are the *Eating Energy* criteria for assessing nutritional value.

Overview: The Eating Energy 12 Optimal Nutrition Factors©

1. **Quality:** *Does the food or diet provide the highest quality food sources and get them on the plate?*

2. **Digestion:** *Will the food(s) digest well?*
3. **Assimilation/Humanization:** *Can we assimilate the food after we digest it and can the liver process it into "self"?*
4. **Bio-Availability (Low stress):** *Is the food or meal mostly low-stress, or are there high-stress foods resulting in a loss of vitality? In other words, does the food/diet provide more energy than it takes the body to process it?*
5. **Balance of the macro-nutrients (protein, carbohydrate, and fat):** *Will the food provide and maintain our balance of macro-nutrients and support a balanced hormonal response to the meal?*
6. **Complete, balanced micro-nutrients (vitamins, minerals):** *How rich is the food in vitamins and minerals?*
7. **Enzymes:** *Are there an abundance of living enzymes in the food or meal, or is it a "dead" food?*
8. **pH (acid/alkaline balance):** *Does the diet support the proper acid activity cycle and alkaline reserve of the blood and tissues?*
9. **Fiber:** *Is there adequate fiber provided for proper absorption of nutrients and proper transit time of food through the intestines?*
10. **Water Content:** *Is the food or diet water-bearing as opposed to dehydrating?*
11. **Detoxification:** *Does the food contribute to the body's toxic burden, or does it assist in the cleansing of cellular wastes?*
12. **Bio-energy – The life factor:** *Does the meal or diet impart vitality, (ch'i, or qi energies) to the person's electromagnetic field? Our cells receive nutrients via an electrical charge. If a food depletes that charge, the body must add energy to the food. If the food carries vitality, it serves the body with ease and contributes to the electrical and electromagnetic activities of health.*

The Weight Is Over will not go deeper into these issues, which are covered fully in *Eating Energy.* This book will use these factors as a sorting mechanism to establish the beneficial and detrimental foods for your consideration. Each macro-nutrient category has a full array of possibilities. When we emphasize the beneficial foods and minimize the detrimental, we support our health. Rather than spend a lot of time analyzing specific foods, *The Weight Is Over* will teach how to arrange our meals so they meet the 12 Optimal Nutrition Factors. Thus one food can compensate for another, less-than-optimal food and provide a positive impact on the Vitality. This will provide a broader range of foods that will appeal to more people. If you are interested in dietary and nutritional perfection (virtually an oxymoron), that information is covered in the more-detailed *Eating Energy.*

The 12 Optimal Food Factors bring a powerful dimension to your *The Weight Is Over* Program. They provide the opportunity for you to experience the best of the best. For many people, these health-enhancing foods are the difference between health and disease, and ultimately the difference between life and death. This book will teach you how to seek out the best foods so you can build a truly optimal state of dietary health.

CHAPTER TWO

Successful Fat-Loss Thinking

Ye shall know the truth and the truth shall set you free. - St. John

Currently, in the natural health field, information is presented from one of two viewpoints. Either you get unsubstantiated ideas that may or may not be very beneficial, or you get hard scientific facts that may or may not be beneficial. There are virtues and fallacies to both sides.

> *There are more things in heaven and earth, Horatio, than are dreamt of in your philosophy.*
> – Wm. Shakespeare

If people lean toward an anti-scientific approach (because science doesn't know everything and often looks in the wrong place) then they will believe the stories, the claims, or the interpretation of facts, even if there are no studies to prove it. Industries are built on such claims. The theory sounds good and many people choose to believe it. Often, some people can benefit from the unsubstantiated theory. On the other hand, many people can be misled by a good, but unproveable story. *Caveat emptor* ("Buyer beware.")

In the other camp are the hard scientists. They are all molecules and equations. "If it's not a proven fact, then it's not valid," is their creed. Scientific facts are expanding the nutritional horizons at a rapid rate with new and exciting knowledge that provides a better understanding of how to be healthy. Yet, as a general rule, much of what Science laughs at today will be scientific fact in twenty years. This often occurs because the tunnel vision necessary to delve deeply into a subject omits the broader perspective.

Thus, we can laugh a little at both sides and their shortcomings. We can also benefit from both sides if only we can have the insight to pick and choose the gems and discard the rocks.

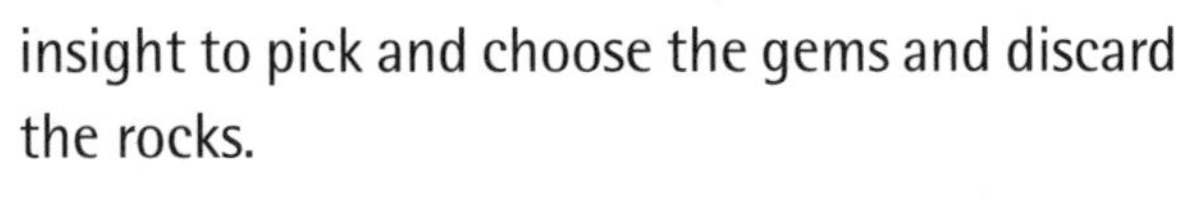

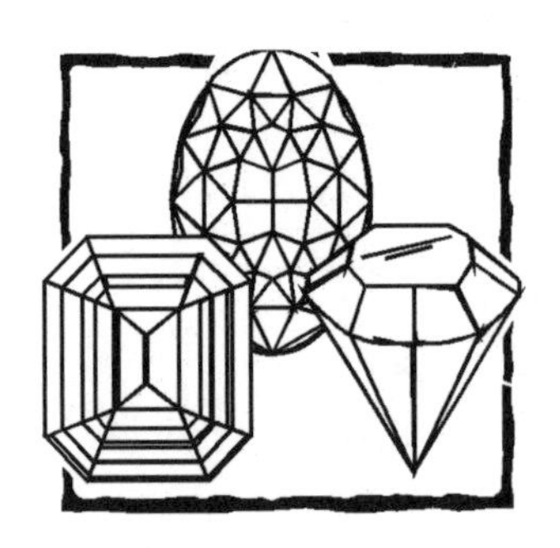

The insights presented in *The Weight Is Over* will pay respect to both views and take the best of both camps. Modern discoveries are tempered with "ancient wisdom." This way, we won't be mislead or overlook the jewels right in front of our noses. We won't be the first or the last. We won't follow fad after fad in an elusive search for help. Instead, we'll help ourselves to the best of the best.

The Ancient Wisdom

The phrase "ancient wisdom" conjures up the great truths and wisdom of the ages. You might wonder if it is the sayings of wise sage or the platitudes of a guru sitting on a mountain explaining the riddle of life. Despite the mystique of its name, the "ancient wisdom" is really quite simple. It's based more on horse sense and practicality than on lofty philosophies.

Nutritional truth is often found between the hard science "facts" and the ancient wisdom "sense."

I believe that nutrition is basically simple. It's the *study* of nutrition that becomes so complex. What makes this book necessary is that we must first undo some mistakes and correct a few problems before we can get back to that state of grace where our adaptive, balancing mechanism can take care of us the way Nature intended. Even though the mistakes are complex, we'll use the sounding board of the "ancient wisdom" to keep our bearings and simplify what we do. Ancient wisdom is the simple, common-sense question "why" that seeks the *cause* of a symptom; and the simple question "Where in Nature do we see the basis for a nutritional fact or theory?"

The "ancient wisdom" is a phrase I use to get in touch with the Natural Laws that govern our health. Don't let the word "Law" scare you. Nature is not a rigid, domineering overlord. In fact, flexibility is a keynote of Nature. If we know about the Natural Laws, and understand basically how our bodies are designed to work, it is easy to do the right things for our health. When we abide within the "ballpark" of Natural Law, we get to enjoy the game. If we live outside those laws, then symptoms of illness and death are the inevitable results.

Ancient wisdom is the often-overlooked common sense principle that baffles the experts.

Ancient wisdom is based on a simple premise that Nature is the function of a balanced system. Left alone, most of the time, everything works well. Deviations from Nature are controlled by "survival of the fittest". "Survival of the fittest" is a phrase that defines what a person suffers when deviating outside of Nature's parameters or standing too long outside the ballpark. The erratic fish soon becomes prey. The sluggish deer soon becomes the wolf's dinner. The overfed, undernourished human being soon becomes obese and develops chronic degenerative diseases.

Here is an example of recent "Ancient Wisdom." Granny says that to get your strength back after a bout of flu, you need chicken soup. Why does she say that? Her grandmother said it and she's seen it work. Why does it work? Granny doesn't know. Today's science recently discovered that the minerals and nucleoproteins in the chicken broth directly replenish the exhausted nutrition reserves and speed the completion of the immune system's development of antibodies. In this instance, ancient wisdom equals scientific fact. As long as we use the "chicken" that Granny used (free range, no hormones added, no-antibiotics added, "roostered," happy chicken), we should get the same results.

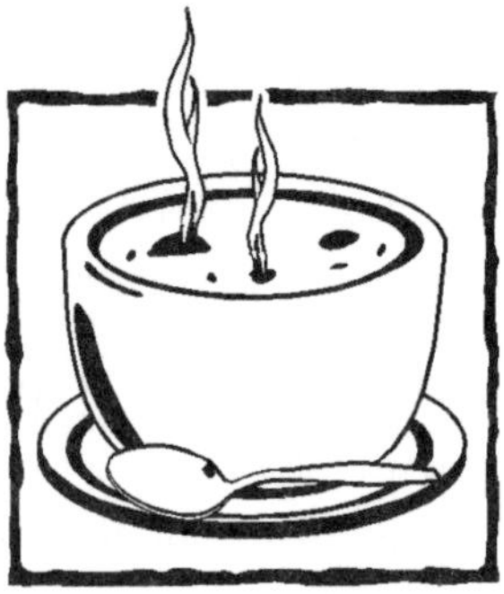

Why do carnivore animals eat grass when they are ill? Eating grass is instinctive, ancient wisdom. Is it the minerals, the chlorophyll, the enzymes, the pH (acid/alkaline balance), or the water? The reason is yet for science to discover. In the meantime, eating grass is instinctive and it often works. It even works for humans as exemplified when a glass of wheat-grass juice or barley-grass powder wards off an ailment.

Here's a question for you. Is it women's destiny to bear children, then get osteoporosis and die like many in the medical profession tell us, or does the ancient wisdom present another model of strong bone-density throughout life? Are there examples of elderly women with strong bones? If so, how do they do it? What if they lived before estrogen replacement? This was the topic of an essay I wrote called "Osteoporosis, the Preventable Disease," (*Women's Health Discourses,* Tips, 1990) and I bet you have a good idea what the conclusions are.

The ancient wisdom helps us be wiser and make right choices regarding our health.

The Ancient Wisdom will help us avoid being beguiled by partial truth. It will help us be skeptical when that position is wise; and it will help us embrace "new" concepts more readily when we see their deep roots. It will make us think for ourselves. It keeps us in the ballpark of Natural Law.

An example where "reserve" rather than "rush-in" might be wise arises with the modern-day health claims about the synthetic oil, Olestra, which made the jump from test tube to the human food supply in 1996. This product is being marketed to people who are irrationally afraid of fat. They are being told that now there is a fat that fries their food, but can't enter the bloodstream. A fat-fearful public might think that this is a health breakthrough. Here is an excerpt from the natural health literature that offers a glimpse of ancient wisdom:

> *Created by food chemists' research in linking esters with alcohols, Olestra™ was discovered to be a polyester too large to pass through the intestines and unable to be broken down by enzymes. The food industry now can make fat-free products that are fried, taste like the real thing, but do not deliver fat into the body.*
>
> *Olestra has nutritional side effects. It absorbs fat-soluble vitamins. When Olestra is eaten, the person will lose Vitamin A that prevents flu and protects the intestinal mucosa; will lose Vitamin D needed for assimilation of calcium; will lose Vitamin E needed to protect the heart from the effects of free radicals; and will lose Vitamin K needed for blood clotting. Olestra also absorbs carotenoids, the beneficial phytochemicals in green leafy vegetables and carrots. Carotenoids, rich in anti-oxidants, are more than 500 nutrients from plants that keep the immune system healthy and prevent cancer, heart disease, and eye diseases. They help prevent rancidity or oxidation of essential fatty acids in the body, and thus help lower the incidence of free-radical damage.*
>
> *Beyond the potentially devastating nutritional depletions, Olestra causes some physical side effects including loose stools and rapid transit of food material through the intestine resulting in a loss of other nutrients. In some cases, Olestra causes anal leakage. These symptoms could be Nature's way of telling people that this fake fat doesn't belong in our bodies.*
>
> *The primary use for Olestra is to make useless foods seem guiltless. Now such "important" foods as chocolate ice cream, brownies, French fries, cookies, cakes, chicken fried steak,*

and pie, can be eaten without deep fryer fat and even less nutrition getting into the body.

In an era when people are starving for balanced essential fatty acids, $200,000,000 dollars of research brings us the ability to feel guiltless about junk food. Olestra may trick our taste buds, but deep down we know that we cannot trick Mother Nature. Eventually, the nutrition-depleting aspects of a pretend diet will send people to the doctor with chronic degenerative diseases.

Based on the ancient wisdom, clinical experience, and an inherent mistrust of highly processed, chemically processed, and scientifically altered foods; a reasonable doubt must exist. "Look before we leap" is the best position on this issue at this time. Despite the bandwagon claims, there are some fundamental issues we must satisfy. This is how the ancient wisdom will help guide us into making moderate decisions and hopefully help us avoid making serious mistakes.

The Ancient Wisdom will also help us separate "therapies" from "lifestyle". We'll ask the question, "Where in Nature did people or animals do something?" For example, let's say that someone tells us we should only drink distilled water and nothing else. Chances are this person is a distiller salesperson, but let's ask our question, "Where in Nature do people or animals drink only distilled water?" Here we must look to cultures that drink only pure rainwater or to creatures that drink only dew. We should also look at cultures that drink other waters such as glacier water, spring water, well water, tap water, and so forth. Then, we can decide if this is what Nature intends.

Periodically in this book, we'll examine the Ancient Wisdom to provide either a broader perspective or a narrower frame of reference on a subject. In past generations, people lived more instinctively. Ancient Wisdom provides us with clues to understanding the present with common sense and knowledge from trial and error. We must learn from the past to build a beneficial future.

- The Pueblo Indians knew that maize meal tortillas became more nutritious when charcoal was added. It sounds crazy until Science shows that the carbon structure of charcoal renders more protein from the corn – a nutrient they obviously needed in greater quantities for health.

- Why did Indians in Texas grind up unappetizing hackberries for food? A scientific analysis of their diet showed a calcium deficiency that hackberries completed.

The Ancient Wisdom keeps us from losing touch with common sense. It helps us identify nutritional myths. One common sense example: did anyone ever tell you to not eat eggs or else you'd get cholesterol in your blood? Let's apply Ancient Wisdom. "Where in Nature do we eat a complex food and then find it in our blood?" If we eat oysters, do we get *oyster* in our blood? If we eat bananas, can we draw 5 cc of blood and find banana? Of course not! Our foods are broken down to sugars, amino acids, and lipids: the three macro-nutrient categories of carbohydrate, protein, and fat. Foods also render vitamins, minerals and nutrient factors; but they don't enter the blood as complex molecules like oyster, banana, or cholesterol.

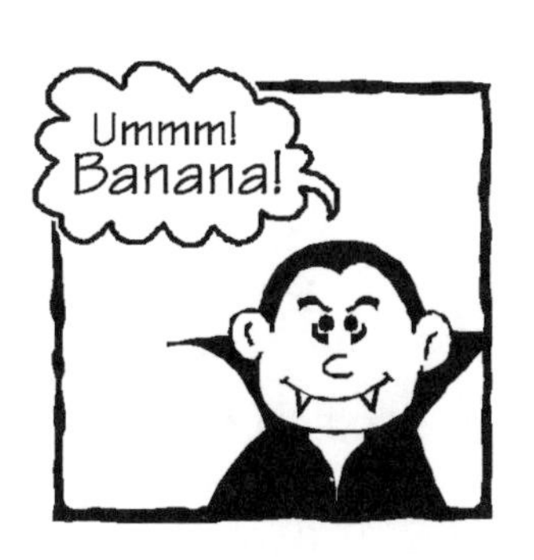

So what happens to the cholesterol in an egg? It's broken down to lipids, simple fat molecules that the body uses for thousands of beneficial processes. The bloodstream gets lipids or fatty acids. The bloodstream does not get cholesterol from one of Nature's nutritious foods. [In Nature, the egg comes from a free-range, natural-food fed chicken; not a caged, force-fed, artificial light bird given hormones, antibiotics, and artificial coloring agents to stain pale yolks yellow.] Further, do people or animals that eat a lot of natural eggs in their natural culture have elevated cholesterol? The answer is, "No."

Why would "knowledgeable" people perpetuate a lie? One answer is that they lost touch with the whole picture – a picture that includes the ancient wisdom. They jumped on a bandwagon, or slanted facts to suit a personal philosophy. Whatever the reason, you and I want to think before we act, look before we leap.

Finally, the ancient wisdom will show us how the processed foods of the industrial revolution are destroying our health and how simple adjustments (which I call "shifts right") in our diets can make a dramatic difference in our weight and overall health. Do we all go back to Nature and swing naked in the trees? As fun as that might sound to some people, of course not. We need to take the best of what the industrial revolution brings us and discard the shortcuts that are killing us. We need to apply technology to bring out the very best of health. To do this, we need to understand the care and feeding of our bodies so they can work their best and provide us the opportunity for a full and varied life, without chronic degenerative disease.

Fat Loss, Not Weight Loss

Because of the many people who are overweight, the issue of "weight loss" is a constant preoccupation. The material in this book is not geared toward weight loss as much as it's geared toward fat loss. This is what overweight people really want – fat loss, not weight loss. Why this distinction? Because it is the excess fat that is ruining a person's health and appearance, not weight. Here's the story.

The body's weight comes from bones, organs, muscles, water, and fat. We don't really want to lose bone to reduce weight, neither do we want to lose muscle. Losing water weight doesn't alter the fat to muscle ratios in the body, and water weight can quickly return. Removing a lung or kidney will help reduce weight, but it's not a viable way to optimize weight.

Unfortunately, many weight loss programs also cause muscle mass to be lost. When this happens, the muscle's fat-burning potential is lost with the weight. Low calorie diet plans, fasting, or cleanses that focus on fruit or fruit drinks also run the risk of muscle loss along with fat loss.

The real goal is to lose fat.

Some of the "I lost 40 pounds" stories are nothing more than water weight loss, which does not change fat-to-muscle ratios – they are not genuine fat-loss stories. Poundage was lost, but to genuinely improve health, the body needs to have access to fat for energy and burn it. The right way to lose weight is to burn fat and increase muscle so that when a person's weight is correct, there is the muscle mass to continue burning fat and help maintain the optimal weight. Of course, the side effect of this is a wonderful, lean, sexy physique. If that no longer appeals to you, the other side effect is better health and vitality.

This is why many weight loss programs must first know the amount of body fat a person has compared to lean muscle mass. The successful program will decrease fat and increase muscle. This means that there may not be a lot of initial weight loss because a person might lose a pound of fat and gain a pound of muscle, but, as the program continues, fat loss accelerates and health improves.

Fat loss and improved health are exactly what this program accomplishes when your diet supports the proper hormonal activities in your body. We simply set the stage for the body to move back into its optimal blueprint. Rather than tell you what not to eat to cut back on dietary fat, **this book will tell you what and how to eat to unleash your body's powerful balancing mechanism**. Then all you have to do is let Nature take its course. Of course, there are many things you should not eat, but coincidentally, they are things that also undermine your health. Here is an opportunity to create a state of vitality that is ten times more enjoyable than eating your favorite junk food. All it takes is a little time.

Change is life's characteristic. Commit to making perpetual positive changes and go with the flow! When we cooperate with Natural Law, the rewards are profound.

Many diet plans attempt to manipulate the body to perform a certain way. Perhaps many nutritionists have gone too deep into the trees and can't find the forest. We've gotten so myopic examining the nuts and bolts of metabolism that the whole machine has become a blur. Let's first restore our nutritional vision and see how simply and effectively our body's "health machinery" works.

Consider Nature's model of humans living a full and varied, active life; then gently passing on during sleep at the end of the road. In the nutrition field, we are inundated with the research showing that what we eat and how we eat it can prevent and reverse chronic, degenerative disease. Nutrition holds the answer to our general state of well being — our quality and quantity of life.

Biochemical Individuality — An Overlooked Principle

For me, part of the joy of writing this book is to present overlooked common-sense principles as well as to dispel myths that block your nutritional freedom. Your *biochemical individuality* (the scientific basis of the uniqueness of every individual) is an overlooked principle that looms large in both nutritional and medical arenas. This universal truth is a primary reason that Western Medicine has struggled with its approach of standardization (to put all people into the same test tube) and a reason that the Naturopathic and nutritional approaches to health have often been successful when all else fails.

Each person is biochemically unique. You are as unique as your fingerprints, as unique as your DNA, as unique as your voice and brainwaves.

The uniqueness of every individual explains why so much nutritional research is misapplied when using the concept of "one size fits all". The axiom, "one person's meat is another person's poison" exemplifies the ancient wisdom of this concept of biochemical individuality.

Let's have a moment's fun with a "sacred cow" of nutritionists. How about when someone parrots the phrase, "Everyone needs 8 glasses of water a day"? Do you ever wonder if this is true for a child, an athlete running 20 miles a day, a person whose diet is mostly raw fruit and vegetables, an international pilot breathing dry air for 12 hours, a person with kidney disease? Don't you know, deep down inside, that optimal water intake is not the same for everyone?

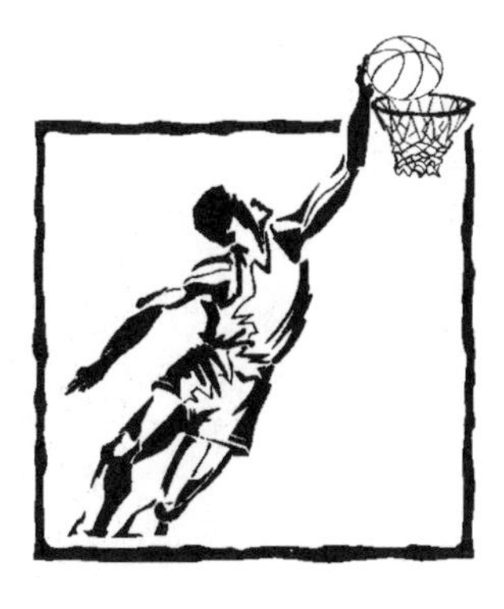

Do we dare take a shot at the phrase, "All men are created equal?" Have you ever seen all men to be equally endowed – mentally, emotionally, spiritually, physically? I don't know about you, but I don't cause hearts to throb the way Tom Cruise and Brad Pitt do (at least not anymore!). I can't fly through the air to dunk a basketball and "be like Mike."

Our nutritional needs are as individual as our fingerprints. They are as unique as our DNA. No two people are exactly the same. Of course, there are many similarities among all people such as the need for air, water, touch, love, light, and food; but there are vast differences as well. As for nutrition, *viva la difference.* The differences in metabolic processes are the defining considerations and play a critical role in weight loss and optimal health.

Hundreds of books have been written to tell us what is the right diet for human beings – vegetarian, carnivore, low fat, raw foods, high protein, high carbohydrate, basic food groups, fruit for breakfast, *et au nauseum.* Most of these books have suffered under the erroneous premise that "what works for one person works for all people." Even worse, many authors have made the assumption that if the theory *sounds* good, it must be true. This is precisely why so many people have tried an eating plan and failed; only to run to another "one size fits all" plan and try again.

The correct answer to the all pervasive question, "What is the right diet for human beings?" is this: "It's none of the above!" The right diet is what supports metabolic balance (hormonal balance) and brings forth optimal health **for the individual.** This right diet varies according to the person's metabolic profile, time of life, gender, lifestyle, geography, and genetics. This means that even Mike can't "be like Mike" now that he's retired from basketball. Why? His lifestyle has changed. Golf does not have the same stamina requirements as the final two-minutes in the National Basketball Association.

For other examples: in the tropics, year-round fruit works well, but in the Arctic, a diet higher in fat is better. Young people can burn more carbohydrates than older people can. Athletes need more protein than sedentary people do. Contrary to popular belief and practice, teenagers do not need more pizza and sodas than adults do.

The Nutritional Ballpark

Biochemical individuality doesn't mean we have to create five billion individual diet plans. Just a few categories will get most people into the ballpark where they can refine their approach based on their individual needs. Our bodies were made to survive in many harsh environments and under many nutritional handicaps. Fortunately – "saving grace" to the rescue – we only have to get into the right "ballpark" to enjoy the game. Once in the right ballpark, our bodies take over and make our nutrition work for us. The secret is to get in the park! This book shows you how to get into the right ballpark. Where you sit in the stands or when you get to bat is based on your goals and how well you practice the nutritional principles.

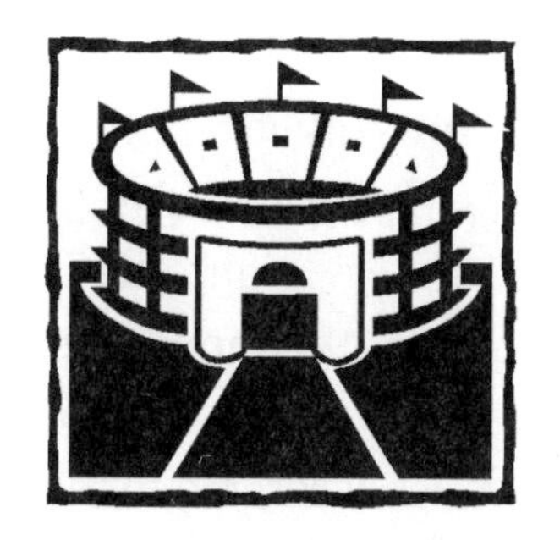

When we get the key factors in our diet right, there is actually a lot of slack in what we do on a daily basis. Once we determine the big dietary factors and live within those broad parameters, and once we choose the foods that provide the necessary small components, we have the freedom from worrying about what we eat all the time. We can live and achieve other goals of human endeavor.

I have shied away from any dietary philosophy that makes me think about what *not* to eat all the time. I call these approaches the "worried sick" diets because people following them become overly

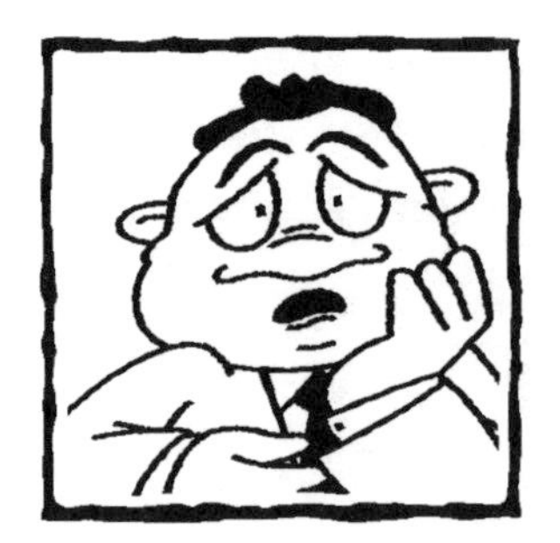

preoccupied with eating and fearful of eating something "wrong." I much prefer dietary freedom based on responsibility to maintain our bodies and the varied activities that freedom allows.

The Veritable Cornucopia of Nutrition

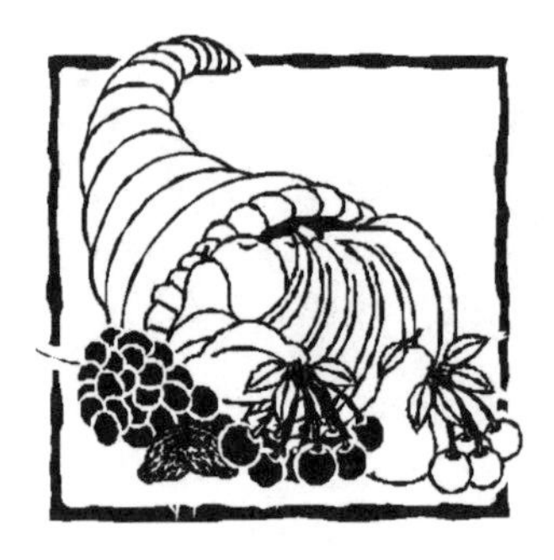

When you pick up a diet book, or hear about a nutrition regimen, does it address **all** the criteria of dietary health? If not, then you will be denied the whole picture and your overall health will suffer. You'll be left outside the ballpark fence staring at the replay monitor. The right diet will contain these general criteria, which specifically apply to proper weight management. It will provide the body the right amounts or ratios of:

1. The macro-nutrients (protein, fat, carbohydrate)
2. The micro-nutrients (vitamins, minerals, trace minerals, nutrient complexes, alkaline reserve)
3. Water (the right amount of the right kind)
4. Living enzymes (raw foods)
5. Fiber

The Weight Is Over Program addresses all these criteria. Beyond these fundamental issues, this book will teach you to use the high quality foods in each of the three macro-nutrient categories!

The five "spinning plates" listed above are five of the *12 Optimal Nutrition Factors* listed in the previous chapter and explained in detail in *Eating Energy*. These five Optimal Nutrition Factors are the most important dietary considerations to a person losing weight. They are presented here for you to start considering your diet as it **was** and get a glimpse of how wonderful it **is** as you introduce *The Weight Is Over* principles.

The dynamic of life called vitality occurs when all the nutritional factors spin correctly together.

When these elements are in the right proportions for your individual metabolism, you will experience:

- A healthy appetite (lack of cravings)
- A beneficial hormonal balance (the basis of optimal weight and health)
- An effective digestion system
- Effective assimilation of nutrients
- Effective elimination of digestive by-products
- Effective detoxification of metabolic and environmental waste products
- Strong energy metabolism (and the myriad benefits that come from living in harmony with your body's inherent blueprint (memory, energy, libido.)

Beyond the basic benefits, when all the nutritional components spin together, there is a magic – an intangible factor – that occurs. There is a synergism that the whole is greater than the sum of the parts. It is the dynamic vitality of the joy of living that can best be described as "full of wonder" or *wonderful!* Somewhere between bliss and ecstasy is a positive, enthusiastic, loving, helpful, joyous, balanced, clear, effective, appreciative, tolerant, peaceful, active, relaxed state of natural wonder that is the desirable home of human life-experience.

Dr. Roger Williams, the eminent nutritional researcher, established the *Law of Biochemical Individuality* in 1956. Today, it is a scientific fact. In broad terms, men's nutrition is different from women's. Young people need different nutrition than the elderly. However, beyond broad parameters, people have vastly different metabolic profiles that require different ratios of nutrients to function optimally. Basic needs, such as air and water, are universal. All people need food, but food requirements for optimal health and weight vary according to numerous conditions. Further, food choices can allow and accelerate the fat-burning processes.

In the old days, people's instincts helped. If more fat was needed to balance the metabolism, then the person sought out and ate more fat. If more protein was needed, that's what the person sought. Today, our instincts are often warped due to the dramatic change in dietary patterns. The Industrial Revolution's impact on the Earth's food supply has caused a major impact on our nutrition, particularly due to the ready availability of altered edible matter, especially refined, denatured carbohydrates (sugars, snacks, soft drinks) and altered fats. Now, we can easily flood our systems with "cheap fuel frequently" to make up for the "quality fuel" that the right diet would bring. This is why *quality* is more important than *quantity* where human nutrition is concerned. A scientific, laboratory test is needed to learn the right dietary ballpark for each individual, because it will see through the warped instincts and rationalizations. It can get us a ticket to the right ballpark.

We all know that weight-loss programs work for some people, but not for others. For example: Mary lost 40-pounds eating hard-boiled eggs and pickled pig's feet, but Tom gained 40 pounds trying the same diet. Wisely, we have learned to be mistrustful and skeptical, because any "recipe book" approach is not individualized to our metabolism and may not work. When we approach a program, we come with both doubt and hope that we'll be the lucky lottery winners and *the program will work for us!* It is important to take the guesswork out of nutrition and base our decisions on facts. A lab test can provide us with irrefutable facts about our bodies' glucose metabolism, which, as we will soon discover, is the basis for our inherent fat gain/fat loss mechanisms.

A simple laboratory test, combined with body measurements, can define what ballpark a person needs to be in to burn fat and improve health.

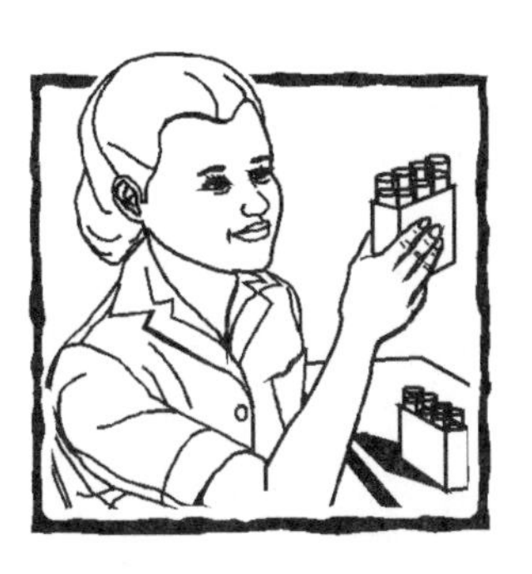

This information is a nutritional breakthrough! There is now a scientific way to understand the key weight-loss factor in your metabolic processes. This key factor determines fat-weight loss as well as helps modulate energy and other important functions such as blood pressure, immune function and inflammatory processes. What a tremendous blessing! The same method of eating that will help a person lose weight will also promote the best of health. This is true nutrition – not how to manipulate our bodies, but how to nourish ourselves back to optimal performance.

To avoid oversimplification, let me clarify that the key metabolic pathway in weight gain accounts for 90% of the reasons that people store fat. We are not addressing obesity as a result of thyroid dysfunction, food allergies, and cellular toxicity. The book, *Your Liver – Your Lifeline* (Tips, 1986), delves into these other elements and their nutritional solutions. People who have additional fat weight as a result of those other reasons also have other clear symptoms – low basal metabolism, severe fatigue, bloating after eating, goiters, and so forth.

As you seek to improve your health with nutrition – both dietary and supplementary – *always remember that you are unique*. Ultimately your diet and supplement regimen **is best when it's based on a custom-designed approach**. Now, let's claim the overlooked principle of biochemical individuality and apply it to our personal nutritional quest. You and I have unique biochemistries and unique metabolic processes. We must first address our uniqueness to find the right diet. It only makes sense. The eating plan needed by a 300-pound football guard must be different than the thin fashion model's. A simple lab test, the FitTest, helps us define the macro-nutrient parameters that will help unleash the health within. The FitTest is described in the following chapter.

CHAPTER THREE

The FitTest™ – The Weight Is Over

The great aim of culture [is] the aim of setting ourselves to ascertain what perfection is, and to make it prevail. - Matthew Arnold

Your Key To Fat Loss

The FitTest™ is a first – a groundbreaking lab analysis that provides key insights into how to eat to lose weight. Basically, analysis of the FitTest information will show you the combination to foods' ability to unlock your fat-burning mechanism!

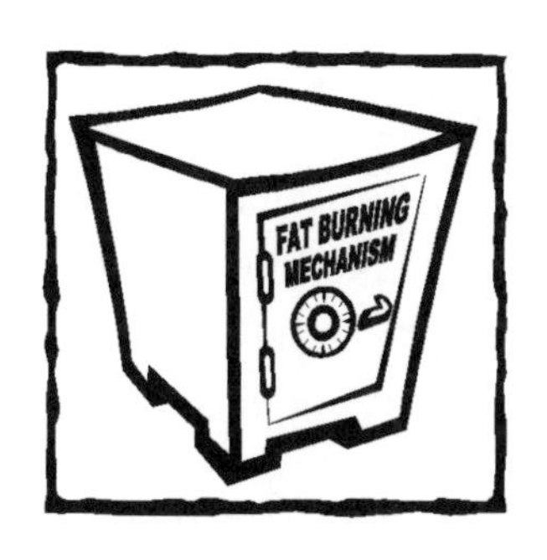

In more specific terms, here's what the FitTest is about. It is a non-invasive, urinary test (collection) that can reveal the tendency to hyper-insulinemia (excessive insulin hormone), which is linked with insulin resistance and the fat-storage mechanism in your body. Conducted by one of this nation's premier metabolic laboratories, Metametrix Clinical Laboratories, this test provides major insights on how to unlock the body's fat burning mechanism for weight loss, as well as establish hormonal balance for optimal health.

Please note that no other tests are conducted – not alcohol abuse, not drug screening. This is a completely confidential test that looks at only one thing – microalbumin – and then your specimen is destroyed.

Extensive worldwide research has proven relationships between the presence of micro-albumin in the urine and insulin-resistance, kidney problems, cardiovascular risk, diabetes, visceral fat and glucose intolerance. Published studies conducted in the United States, Japan, and China established the interrelations between micro-albumin in the urine, excessive insulin, diabetes, altered fat ratios in the blood, insulin-resistance and excessive fat. All of these scientific issues are related to obesity.

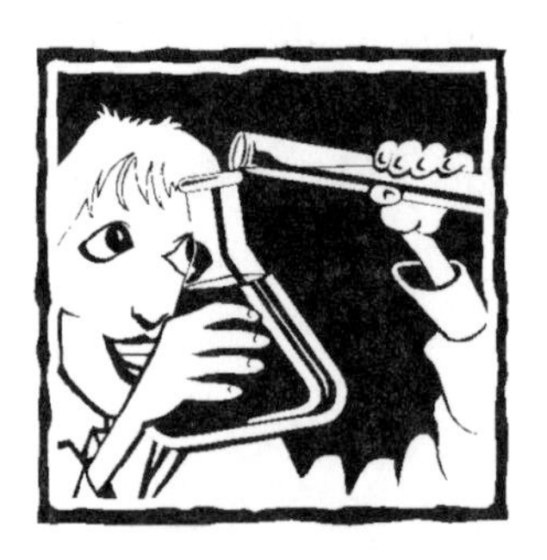

The FitTest is creating a revolution in both nutrition as well as weight-loss science because it provides you with insights into dietary parameters regarding macro-nutrient balance. This balance of protein to carbohydrate to fat is your powerful ally to activate the hormone, *glucagon,* the fat-burning hormone. Since the FitTest can reveal exactly where dietary improvements are needed, it is an empowering nutritional breakthrough that can help you improve your health and lose weight.

Dr. J. Alexander Bralley (the chief scientist and director of MetaMetrix Laboratories) developed the nutritional applications of FitTest. When combined with his pioneering nutritional insights, the FitTest provides a clear picture of the ratios of macro-nutrients (protein, carbohydrate, fat) that will help stop the storage of fat and help burn excess fat, resulting in weight normalization.

With the FitTest results, you can begin to eat to lose weight! While you're losing weight using proper ratios of macro-nutrients, combined with the other key nutritional principles in this book, you can begin to experience a more optimal health and its myriad benefits. All you'll have to do is follow *The Weight Is Over* guidelines regarding the high-quality foods to lose weight and build a healthier future, simultaneously.

Warning! Embarking on a fat-loss diet without laboratory testing is like hiking in the jungle without a guide.

Here's the overview. Your body is designed to run on fuel that is provided by eating. The foods you eat contain three primary nutrients called the macro-nutrients. These macro-nutrients are protein, fat, and carbohydrate (sugars). All foods will fall into one, two, or all three of these macro-nutrient categories.

For example: an egg is mostly a protein food because it is, by percentage, mostly bio-available protein. It also contains a percentage of fat, and a much, much smaller percentage of carbohydrate. Milk is high in carbohydrate (milk sugar), but has substantial fat and protein. It falls into all three categories. Apples are mostly carbohydrate. Avocados and olives are fats. Knowing food-categories helps us plan "balanced" meals. Our individual biochemistry dictates the proper ratios of these macro-nutrients for a balanced hormonal response that can stop storing fat and start burning it. We'll look at food categories in Part Two of this book.

Although glucose (a sugar, the basic carbohydrate) is your cells' primary fuel, your cells actually require a "fuel mix" that includes protein and fat for optimal performance, rather than a pure glucose injection system. Muscle cells prefer to burn fat because it is a longer burning fuel and thus provides the stamina that is a chief concern of the muscles. Beyond meeting your cells' energy requirements, the macro-nutrients cause powerful hormonal responses that control much of the body's metabolism. It's the hormone response that makes a person either store fat, stay the same, or burn fat.

Thus there are three general hormonal responses to the ratios of macro-nutrient foods that you eat in any meal:

1. The storage of fat mediated by the insulin hormone response

to carbohydrates (excessive protein can also elicit an insulin response),

2. The status quo (no major change because of the balance between the hormones insulin and glucagon in relationship to caloric needs,)

3. The burning of fat mediated by the glucagon hormone response to protein and primed by the presence of essential fatty acids (fat).

Obviously, if your are reading this book to lose weight, you are interested in response number three. So how will you eat to encourage the fat-burning response? The FitTest will show you how.

Food is our most powerful ally in weight loss.

The FitTest documents how your body is responding to the ratios of macro-nutrients you are eating. The test provides insights regarding the master hormone, insulin. By understanding insulin and the resistance to its action at the cellular level, the scientists at MetaMetrix gain the insights to differentiate your dietary approach so you can custom-design an eating plan that can assist your body to return to its optimal weight and more optimal state of health.

The Value of Laboratory Testing

In my practice, laboratory testing is important because it provides irrefutable evidence of biochemical facts. With proper nutritional interpretation, lab tests can reveal keen insights into the body's struggles to maintain balance. Then, an effective individualized program can be designed. The fact that lab work can be repeated at a later time provides the ability to see before and after results. The FitTest allows more precision than a "recipe book approach" in determining the carbohydrate to protein to fat ratios that will unlock the body's access to stored fat. The resulting individualization of the diet means that more people are successful in attaining their fat loss goals in a shorter amount of time.

Over the past ten years, lab tests involving urine, rather than blood, hair, or saliva, have been moving into the forefront of the exciting new health arena called "functional testing." Because urine presents the end-products of cellular metabolism and represents the body's efforts to maintain balance, it is rapidly becoming a premier diagnostic method – one with strong nutritional insights.

Much more than the old fashioned urinalysis that screens for sugar, protein, and infections; functional urinalysis provides keen insights to important metabolic processes including:

- liver function
- adrenal function (DHEA, cortisol)
- insulin resistance (microalbumin)
- immune function (nitric oxide)
- female hormone imbalance (estrodiol, progesterone)
- oxidative stress (lipid peroxides)
- kidney function
- intestinal damage (leaky gut syndrome)
- male hormone imbalance (testosterone)

More tests are being developed, including a test for prostate cancer as well as many nutritional issues.

By identifying what the kidneys are filtering out of the blood and excreting, the doctor or clinical nutritionist can quickly determine the functional status of the organ in question and the nutritional implications. With sophisticated advancements in laboratory testing, the old concept that urine can only reveal kidney function has long given way to the amazing, non-invasive insights of urinary laboratory testing.

Often, the necessary lab tests are very expensive. I so often regret that the truly valuable lab tests are expensive and that people's insurance will not help pay for them because they are investigative or nutritionally-oriented. One solution to that dilemma is to have affordable lab tests interpreted by smart people who can derive deep insights from the results.

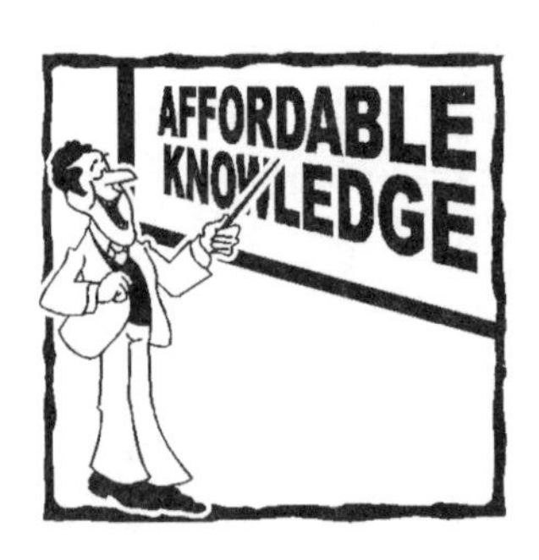

Fortunately, innovative people still have freedom to bring lab tests to the public for self-knowledge – visionaries who want to bring knowledge directly to people, affordably. Now you can see why I am excited about bringing this information to you. I believe that people deserve access to knowledge about their bodies and health. End of soapbox.

The FitTest™ Concept Works For You!

The confusion and misinformation surrounding weight loss is rampant. Over the past five years, a rediscovery of the Natural Laws that govern our health has emerged to challenge the low-fat, low-cholesterol food pyramid "party line" under which America has suffered, growing fatter and fatter each year. This "new" philosophy embraces the ancient wisdom that fat is not the culprit by itself, but that fat, in combination with certain types and amounts of carbohydrate, is the real reason behind the blimping pandemic of obesity that is reaching its chubby little fingers right into our kindergartens. No longer are books like *The Pro-Vita! Plan for Optimal Nutrition* (Tips, 1987) lone voices in the wilderness. There are volumes of scientific evidence and support for proper nutrition and more are emerging every day.

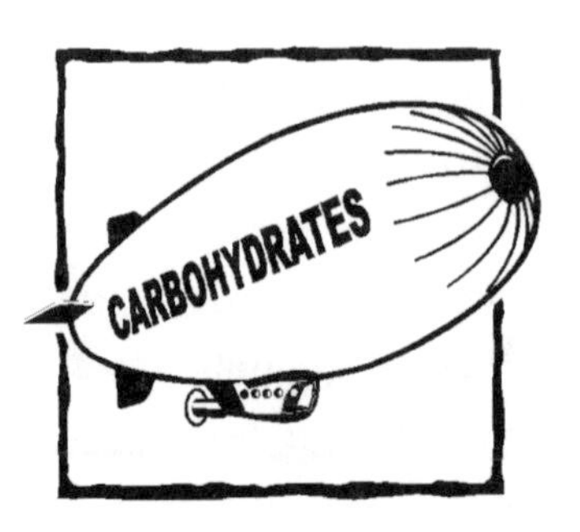

As with all "new" ideas, within the ranks of the supporters of balanced nutrition, there are several schools of thought and approach. Most try to fit everyone into their system without regard for biochemical individuality. These people tell us there is only one ratio of macro-nutrients for all people. Of course, this is not so. With the FitTest, we examine the individual. For the first time in the perpetual battle to lose weight, we have a method to take the confusion and struggle out of losing fat-weight.

The Scientific Basis for the FitTest and The Weight Is Over approach to Fat Loss

For a more in-depth look at the science of the FitTest and how it, along with other data, can be used to better evaluate an individual's diet to stop the unnecessary storage of fat, initiate the fat-burning mechanism, and improve overall health, here are the insights of Dr. Bralley.

Q and A with Dr. J. Alexander Bralley:

Q. *The quest for the optimal diet has been as elusive as the Holy Grail. Conflict, controversy, and confusion are the Three C's everyone encounters when trying to improve their health nutritionally. Why is it so difficult to eat for optimal health?*

A. Dr. Bralley: "There is much confusion in the medical literature as to what constitutes a healthy diet which minimizes and prevents disease. Macro-nutrient intake of protein, carbohydrate, and fat can vary in different populations. Conflicting evidence has accumulated as to what are the most appropriate ratios of these to be consumed to optimize health. This conflict arises due to a model which assumes genetic homogeneity of the population such that each person is the same regarding how their bodies handle macro-nutrient intake.

"It is proposed that a more appropriate and realistic model takes into account genetic diversity and biochemical individuality in regards to hormonal responses to dietary intake. This would give a range of appropriate macro-nutrient ratios which best suit the individual."

Q. *So the key is to have a method that evaluates the expression of a person's genetics as well as tangible evidence (anatomy) of their hormonal response to their diet and lifestyle. Would this not, then, provide better insight into how a person should eat rather than the "one size fits all" approaches so prevalent today?*

A. Dr. Bralley: "Absolutely. The use of urinary microalbumin combined with waist/hip ratio and other personal data can be a useful and accurate means of determining the most appropriate combinations of macro-nutrients which best support a healthful life."

Q. *And that's exactly what* The Weight Is Over *Program does. Before we delve further into the FitTest, will you please discuss the importance of the appropriate diet?*

A. Dr. Bralley: "Certainly. Maintenance of optimal is health is a complicated issue with many factors contributing to it, including genetic predisposition, exercise, environmental factors and diet. Dietary intake is a powerful tool over which humans have control that can influence health. It would be good to know what is the best diet to eat to maintain a healthy life. Researchers have pondered this question for many years with conflicting results. We have the "Food Pyramid" promoted by the American Dietetic Association (ADA) as the prototypical ideal mix of food intake at the same time as we have ketchup classified as a vegetable for school lunch programs. And yet, with all this emphasis on good diet, obesity in Americans has reached epidemic proportions. It has been estimated that 300,000 premature deaths in the U.S. will be caused by obesity related conditions in 1999 and will cost the economy $100 billion."

[Comment: This is because researchers have failed to understand that the **quality** *of a food source is of primary importance to nutrition. School children eat French fries with ketchup and cheese whiz. According to the ADA, this is a balanced meal! It even includes "good wholesome vegetables" in the form of "ketchup". Anyway, sorry for the interruption.]*

"One of the areas in which diet has been understood as having a major effect is in the treatment and prevention of cardiovascular disease. Over 1.5 million Americans have heart attacks each year. For a third of these, it is the first sign of a heart problem. Forty million people in the US have diagnosed heart disease and many more don't know it. High serum cholesterol is found in 80 million Americans and 60 million people have high blood pressure. With these alarming statistics, one would think a good dietary program would be readily available from our medical scientists.

"Yet there is much confusion among the experts as to what exactly constitutes a "healthy diet." In the 1960's Nathan Pritikin championed the very low fat diet for reversal of heart disease. Since fatty deposits were blocking arteries, it would seem logical to eat a low fat diet. Others, including Dr. Dean Ornish, carried this theme further, combining other lifestyle changes to clearly demonstrate that these lifestyle interventions actually reversed heart disease.[1]

"More recently, the low fat, high carbohydrate diet hypothesis has been questioned as new data accumulated indicating that carbohydrate intake and abnormal physiological responses to that intake were causing a problem.[2] Dr. Robert Atkins popularized the low carbohydrate diet concept with his books.[3] Additional authors have picked up on this theme to recommend varying portions of carbohydrate in relation to fat and protein.

"The macro-nutrient (protein, carbohydrate and fat) ratios are now being hotly debated as to which is the best, creating much confusion for the general population. Both camps can point to obvious success stories of people who have gone on their diets and succeeded where other approaches have failed. Both sides point to the dangers in each approach. Eating low amounts of carbohydrate will have a tendency to cause consumption of more saturated fat which, when eaten in excess, has been shown to contribute to heart disease and cancer. On the other hand, a high carbohydrate diet which is low in fat can lead to hyperinsulin responses in individuals who are insulin insensitive.[2] These insulin resistant individuals are at higher risk for heart disease and obesity.[4]"

Q. *We're back to the fact that practically any therapeutic change in diet can temporarily help a person as they pass through a more beneficial ratio of macro-nutrient intake enroute to another imbalance fostered by that therapeutic diet. This is why there are so many examples of people who received benefits after a month or two on a diet, then later, struggle to keep the improvements as that diet takes them to another imbalance. So we really must have an understanding of the individual in order to know what eating plan will bring genuine results, right?*

A. Dr. Bralley: "Right. All of these diets promote the idea that they are healthy ways to eat and lose weight. Many people have experienced success on each dietary program. Yet others have reported failure. In other words, there is no one diet that works for everyone. To complicate issues, most obesity related research and treatment is predicated on the concept that weight loss occurs only if the total calories consumed is less than the total calories burned by the individual. But research is beginning to question this postulate.[5, 6]

"Newer models of obesity are starting to take into account the genetic uniquenesses of people. The details of what is happening during fat gain are beginning to be understood in light of individualized response to macro-nutrient intake. This individualized physiological response is helping to explain the increasing prevalence of obesity and its relationship to health maintenance.

"Research conducted by Gerald Reaven, M.D., at Stanford University School of Medicine has demonstrated a variation in the population in the responsiveness to a carbohydrate load. In about 25% of the normal healthy, non-obese population, there is a genetic tendency to secrete excessive amounts insulin when carbohydrates are eaten. About 50% of the population have a normal response and another 25% produce low amounts of insulin.[7] This range of physiological responsiveness has been viewed as explaining an important part of why people respond differently to varied macro-nutrient content diets.[8] To help clarify the importance of this point, an examination of what happens when one eats a meal is necessary."

Q. *You mean the hormonal response to food intake?*

A. Dr. Bralley: "Yes. Food consumption elicits a complex response in the human body. The task of converting the raw materials of our diet into useable compounds involves many different processes. First, the food must be broken down in the digestive tract. Since food is composed of many different compounds, the digestion and breakdown process itself is not simple, requiring a concentrated acid content in the stomach and multiple enzyme systems to reduce the food compounds to molecules small enough to be absorbed into the bloodstream. The bulk of this digested food goes directly to the liver for further processing. Fat molecules and the amino acids from protein are initially utilized for structural, functional and metabolic support of the system. Any excess is stored as fat. The carbohydrate portion of a meal is initially used to generate energy for the cells. Glucose, the final breakdown product of carbohydrates, circulates in the blood to contact each cell of the body. Insulin is secreted by the pancreas when it senses this rise in blood glucose. Glucose requires this insulin molecule in order to enter the cell. This is the case for all tissues except the eyes, kidneys, and nerves. Once glucose enters the cell, it is metabolized to produce energy for cellular function.

"Since the cell cannot store glucose in any appreciable amounts, this process must continue on an ongoing basis. Between meals, the liver can regulate blood glucose levels by breaking down glycogen, a short-term storage form for glucose. If there is still excess glucose available from the meal which can not be utilized by cells or converted to glycogen, this excess is converted to fat and stored for potential future use."

Q. *So, apart from the old idea that excessive fat intake causes obesity, we now have the evidence that excessive dietary carbohydrate intake causes an excessive insulin response which, in turn, causes fat storage. Is this, then, the premier cause of obesity?*

A. Dr. Bralley: "In part, but lets discuss *Syndrome X.* Dr. Reaven and his colleagues have demonstrated that approximately 25% of healthy non-obese individuals in the US secrete excess amounts of insulin in response to a carbohydrate load. Apparently, these individuals have tissues that, for one reason or another, have become resistant to the effects of insulin such that they require higher amounts to get glucose inside the cell. If the resistance to insulin worsens, diabetes develops. These insulin-resistant individuals consequently are adversely affected by this increased circulating amount of insulin, a powerful hormone that has deleterious ramifications when present in higher amounts in the blood.[9, 10]

"This phenomenon of insulin resistance and its biological ramifications has been referred to as Syndrome X.[7, 11-19] From a clinical standpoint, Syndrome X has been associated with patterns of disease risk: adult onset diabetes, heart disease, hypertension, stroke, polycystic ovary syndrome, breast cancer, hyperuricaemia (elevated serum uric acid), elevated triglycerides, dyslipidemia (low HDL and elevated LDL), rheumatoid arthritis and obesity. People with Syndrome X also tend to store fat in the abdominal area and are often characterized as being "apple shaped."

Q. *So here we have a significant portion of the population that the high-carbohydrate diet is actually leading to an obese and diseased state of health. The FitTest is actually a screening that can save lives! Is this the first point of differentiation of a custom-designed eating plan?*

A. Dr. Bralley: "Of course. In the 25% of individuals with an abnormal insulin response to carbohydrates, it would not be appropriate to recommend a diet with a high percentage of carbohydrate. In these individuals, the affect would be a conversion of the carbohydrates to fat and a tendency to obesity. Conversely the 25% of the population which has a blunted insulin response can do very well on this type of diet. The other 50% of the population are somewhere in between in terms of finding the proper macro-nutrient balance in their diets. The American Heart Association, National Cancer Institute, American Diabetic Association and the American Dietetic Association all recommend a diet with a ratio of percent calories of carbohydrate-protein-fat of 60-20-20.

"This relatively high proportion of carbohydrate would be inappropriate for the Syndrome X person and simply contribute to their health problems, including a tendency to weight gain. The popularized ratio of 40-30-30 would be more appropriate; indeed, in extreme cases, the carbohydrate percentage would best go even lower. With such a range in physiological responsiveness to macro-nutrient intake, it would be useful to identify individual's genetic tendencies in this regard. With a proper identification of each person's unique needs, it would be possible to recommend the best dietary regimen for optimal health and proper weight maintenance."

Q. *Since Syndrome X is so clearly a dangerous position to be in, how can people find out if this applies to them?*

A. Dr. Bralley: "Insulin resistance or Syndrome X is characterized by an elevated fasting insulin level, elevated triglycerides, hypertension, dyslipidemia, hyperuricemia, and an elevated insulin in a two hour oral glucose tolerance test (OGTT). In some cases, the glucose is marginally elevated in the OGTT also. This constellation of indicators represents the classic case of Syndrome X with all the consequent health risks associated with it. People can range in this physiological condition from mild insulin resistance to adult onset diabetes. Identifying one's position on this health continuum is critical to optimal health and development of proper dietary regimes.

"While seeing a doctor and having all of these tests run may be acceptable for some people, this option is not easily available to all. There is another approach one can use to identify one's carbohydrate response. Insulin resistance and its associated dysglycemic or faulty glucose regulation mechanism can also significantly affect kidney function. The kidneys do not require insulin for glucose utilization by its cells. Consequently, the marginal elevations of serum glucose in insulin resistance can over-saturate kidney tissues with glucose, potentially damaging them. The associated hypertension of Syndrome X can also contribute to this degenerative process. Consequently, subtle changes in kidney function have been considered to be signs of a dysglycemic condition in the body."

The FitTest is one of the biggest gifts a weight-challenged person can receive. It's the gift of health renewed.

Q. *Is there a simple way to measure this change in kidney function?*

A. **Dr. Bralley:** "Yes, microalbumin. The kidneys filter the blood, retaining important compounds for body function and excreting excess water and other metabolic waste products. Ordinarily, the kidneys retain serum proteins as the blood passes through the kidney tubules. Slight damage to these tubules can cause a "leaking" of serum proteins, the most abundant of which is serum albumin. This slight excretion of serum albumin in the urine is called microalbumin and has been associated with increased risk for kidney damage in diabetic and hypertensive patients.[20-24]

"Microalbumin has also been associated with the development of insulin resistance.[25-32] Consequently, it could be used as a urinary screening marker for the Syndrome X individual. This, coupled with a waist-to-hip measurement ratio and personal and family history, can provide an accurate assessment of how a person responds to a carbohydrate load. Since insulin-resistant individuals retain fat in the abdominal region, the waist to hip ratio has frequently been used to identify those with this genetic predisposition.[33-35] Because insulin resistance is an inherited genetic trait, it may been seen in the family history as hypertension and/or diabetes.[26]

"The combination of microalbumin data with family history and the anthropometric data of the waist/hip ratio and other pertinent measurements provides a powerful, accurate and cost-effective way of defining one's carbohydrate responsiveness. With this information, the individual can now clearly define what type of macro-nutrient content diet would be most appropriate for optimal health and weight management."

Q. *What insights do the body measurements (anthropometric data) provide?*

A. Dr. Bralley Researcher Rudderman [36, 37, 38] has used this type of data to screen for Syndrome X, particularly the metabolically obese person. The phrase metabolically obese refers to a person who is not obviously obese by body appearance or shape, but is at a high risk for the same diseases such as diabetes or high blood pressure. Because this person is not considered obese to the eye, the disease processes are silently creeping up. The body measurements, along with the urine test, reveal this pattern. This is another reason showing the value of a test such as the FitTest, which examines markers for this type of situation and helps people correct their diets before the Syndrome X pattern can manifest into a disease state.

Note: The references to Dr. Bralleys text are listed at the end of this chapter.

The Weight Is Over, FitTest™ Gift of Health

The United InfoXchange's *The Weight Is Over* program, based on Ideal Health System's FitTest, is a synthesis of body measurements (lean body mass, hip-to-waist ratio, thigh, wrist, and arm measurements), individual health history and risk assessment, and laboratory evaluation of a metabolic marker closely associated with hyperinsulinemia and other health concerns. By evaluating each of these parameters, an individualized pattern of risk emerges which is a clear indicator how assertive a fat-loss intervention program should be. The results of the evaluation can define different classifications of intervention and each individual is placed within one of those categories. The result is *a custom-designed program for maximum results.*

Each program has a specific set of dietary macro-nutrient guidelines, which are presented as a customized eating plan. This plan includes a real "food on the plate" program as well as an optional nutritional supplement program to accelerate the process and help clients reach their goals of fat-loss and improved health more quickly.

HOW TO ORDER YOUR LAB TEST

Ideal Health, International is providing the FitTest™ and InfoXchange's The Weight Is Over Program to the public at a reduced price. Their order line is: 1-800-768-7667.

In about seven days after ordering your FitTest, you will receive your test kit. Full instructions are provided in the kit for both the lab samples and client information. After submitting your urine specimen, questionnaire, and body measurements, within around two weeks you will receive a written report about your results that includes dietary and supplemental insights. Then, you are off and running with a dietary management tool that will reshape your body and your health.

Finally, someone put it all together and raised the standard of excellence in the weight loss arena. Next, we'll focus on the power and freedom that knowledge brings.

- As you wait for FitTest results, you can preview the health of your glucose metabolism with several self-tests in the following chapter.
- Have you ever wondered how or why people become obese? The next section will explain that process and show how to avoid or reverse that process.
- Why is a micro-albumin, insulin-resistance test the perfect determining factor in losing weight and an important facet of being on a health-enhancing diet? To understand that, you'll have to understand the role of insulin in the body and delve into some of the body's biochemistry. This is only slightly technical, and absolutely fascinating! I'm happy to provide that information for those who want a deeper understanding of how their bodies work. I believe that knowledge is power, and since one purpose of this book is to empower people by sharing knowledge, we'll take a look at understanding the metabolic pathway of glucose and insulin, the master hormone. I'll do my best to keep it simple without oversimplifications.

You can begin improving your dietary health with the recommendations in the following chapters. Then, you'll be ready to hit the road running with *The Weight Is Over* program and experience the power of nutrition as you improve your energy, weight, and health!

References:

1. Ornish, D., Program for Reversing Heart Disease. 1990, New York: Ballantine.
2. Reaven, G.M., Do high carbohydrate diets prevent the development or attenuate the manifestations (or both) of syndrome X? A viewpoint strongly against. Curr Opin Lipidol, 1997. 8(1): p. 23-7.
3. Atkins, R., Dr. Atkins New Diet Revolution. 1992, New York, Avon.
4. Laws, A. and G.M. Reaven, Insulin resistance and risk factors for coronary heart disease. Baillieres Clin Endocrinol Metab, 1993. 7 (4): p. 1063-78.
5. Bjorntorp, P., Recent advances in obesity research III. Proceedings of the 3rd International Congress on Obesity. 1980, London, England.
6. Ball, M.F., J.J. Canary, and L.H. Kyle, Comparative effects of caloric restriction and total starvation on body composition in obesity. Ann Intern Med, 1967. 67(1): p. 60-7.
7. Reaven, G.M., Pathophysiology of insulin resistance in human disease. Physiol Rev, 1995. 75(3): p. 473-86.
8. Sears, B., The Zone Diet. 1995, New York: Harper Collins.
9. Mykkanen, L., et al., Low insulin sensitivity is associated with clustering of cardiovascular disease risk factors. Am J Epidemiol, 1997. 146(4): p. 315-21.
10. Lempiainen, P., et al., Insulin resistance syndrome predicts coronary heart disease events in elderly nondiabetic men. Circulation, 1999. 100(2): p. 123-8.
11. Zavaroni, I., et al., Hyperinsulinaemia, obesity, and syndrome X. J Intern Med, 1994. 235(1): p. 51-6.
12. Reaven, G.M., Syndrome X: 6 years later. J Intern Med Suppl, 1994. 736: p. 13-22.
13. Fuh, M.M., et al., Insulin resistance, glucose intolerance, and hyperinsulinemia in patients with microvascular angina. Metabolism, 1993. 42(9): p. 1090-2.
14. Reaven, G.M., Role of insulin resistance in human disease (syndrome X): an expanded definition. Annu Rev Med, 1993. 44: p.121-31.
15. Zavaroni, I., et al., Changes in insulin and lipid metabolism in males with asymptomatic hyperuricaemia. J Intern Med, 1993. 234(1): p. 25-30.
16. Reaven, G.M., The kidney: an unwilling accomplice in syndrome X. Am J Kidney Dis, 1997. 30(6): p. 928-31.

17. Yip, J., F.S. Facchini, and G.M. Reaven, Resistance to insulin-mediated glucose disposal as a predictor of cardiovascular disease. J Clin Endocrinol Metab, 1998. 83(8): p. 2773-6.
18. Reaven, G.M., Insulin resistance and human disease: a short history. J Basic Clin Physiol Pharmacol, 1998. 9(2-4): p. 387-406.
19. Reaven, G.M., Insulin resistance and compensatory hyperinsulinemia: role in hypertension, dyslipidemia, and coronary heart disease. Am Heart J, 1991. 121(4 Pt 2): p. 1283-8.
20. Bianchi, S., R. Bigazzi, and V.M. Campese, Microalbuminuria in essential hypertension. J Nephrol, 1997. 10(4): p. 216-9.
21. Alzaid, A.A., Microalbuminuria in patients with NIDDM: an overview. Diabetes Care, 1996. 19(1): p. 79-89.
22. Bigazzi, R. and S. Bianchi, Microalbuminuria as a marker of cardiovascular and renal disease in essential hypertension. Nephrol Dial Transplant, 1995. 10(Suppl 6): p. 10-4.
23. Parving, H.H., Microalbuminuria in essential hypertension and diabetes mellitus. J Hypertens Suppl, 1996. 14(2): p. S89-93; discussion S93-4.
24. Viberti, G., Prognostic significance of microalbuminuria. Am J Hypertens, 1994. 7(9 Pt 2): p. 69S-72S.
25. Cirillo, M., et al., Microalbuminuria in nondiabetic adults: relation of blood pressure, body mass index, plasma cholesterol levels, and smoking: The Gubbio Population Study. Arch Intern Med, 1998. 158(17): p. 1933-9.
26. Forsblom, C.M., et al., Insulin resistance and abnormal albumin excretion in non-diabetic first- degree relatives of patients with NIDDM. Diabetologia, 1995. 38(3): p. 363-9.
27. Haffner, S.M., et al., Microalbuminuria. Potential marker for increased cardiovascular risk factors in nondiabetic subjects? Arteriosclerosis, 1990. 10(5): p. 727-31.
28. Kim, C.-H., Kim, H-K, Park, et al., Association of microalbuminuria and atherosclerotic risk factors in non-diabetic subjects in Korea. Diabetes Res. Clin. Prac., 1998. 40: p. 191-199.
29. Kuusisto, J., et al., Hyperinsulinemic microalbuminuria. A new risk indicator for coronary heart disease. Circulation, 1995. 91(3): p. 831-7.
30. Mykkanen, L., et al., Microalbuminuria precedes the development of NIDDM. Diabetes, 1994. 43(4): p. 552-7.
31. Mykkanen, L., et al., Microalbuminuria and carotid artery intima-media thickness in nondiabetic and NIDDM subjects. The Insulin Resistance Atherosclerosis Study (IRAS). Stroke, 1997. 28(9): p. 1710-6.

32. Mykkanen, L., et al., Microalbuminuria is associated with insulin resistance in nondiabetic subjects: the insulin resistance atherosclerosis study. Diabetes, 1998. 47(5): p. 793-800.

33. Megnien, J.L., et al., Predictive value of waist-to-hip ratio on cardiovascular risk events. Int J Obes Relat Metab Disord, 1999. 23(1): p. 90-7.

34. Hsieh, S.D. and H. Yoshinaga, Waist/height ratio as a simple and useful predictor of coronary heart disease risk factors in women. Intern Med, 1995. 34(12): p. 1147-52.

35. Hsieh, S.D. and H. Yoshinaga, Abdominal fat distribution and coronary heart disease risk factors in men-waist/height ratio as a simple and useful predictor. Int J Obes Relat Metab Disord, 1995. 19(8): p. 585-9.

36. Ruderman, N., *et al.*, The metabolically obese, normal-weight individual revisited. *Diabetes*, 1998. 47(5): p. 699-713.

37. Ruderman, N.B., S.H. Schneider, and P. Berchtold, The "metabolically-obese," normal-weight individual. *Am J Clin Nutr*, 1981. 34(8): p. 1617-21.

38. Ruderman, N.B., P. Berchtold, and S. Schneider, Obesity-associated disorders in normal-weight individuals: some speculations. *Int J Obes*, 1982. **6**(Suppl 1): p. 151-7.

Disclaimer

The FitTest is not designed to diagnose or treat any disease. The eating plan presented here is not intended for anyone with kidney problems or for pregnant women or women trying to become pregnant.

It is prudent to consult your physician or primary health care provider before starting any weight loss program and this is hereby recommended. People on medications to control cholesterol, blood sugar, or blood pressure should first consult their physicians. Further, people who have had a heart attack within the last six months must consult with their physicians regarding their eating plan before starting on it.

By law, there are certain FDA disclaimers and other legal statements we must present. The Food and Drug Administration has not evaluated the statements you have read. The products, tests, and your results are not intended to diagnose, treat, cure, or prevent any disease.

Ideal Health and Ideal Health International are registered trademarks of Ideal Health Systems, Inc. FitTest is a trademark of Ideal Health Systems, Inc. The Weight Is Over is a trademark of United InfoXchange, Inc. which is used by permission for the purpose of this book only.

CHAPTER FOUR

Self-Tests: Are You Burning Or Building Fat?

Let your food be your medicine, and your medicine be your food. - Hippocrates

Meet Urk Thagstone

This chapter will help us evaluate how healthy our glucose metabolisms are. To understand our circumstances, it helps us to think of our ancestors. Thus, I'll introduce our common ancestor, Urk Thagstone, from the Paleolithic age. Urk, or someone just like him, sits high up on all our family trees. In fact, he probably lived in the trees.

Back then, life was hard. Now, this isn't to say that life isn't hard now, but Urk had to worry about survival issues that are less prominent today, like killing a wooly mammoth for dinner while avoiding becoming his neighbors' dinner. Urk was concerned with day to day survival.

Back then, it was catch as catch can. There was no agriculture. If Urk didn't hunt and catch dinner, or gather an edible plant, he had to survive on the nutrients already in his body from the day before. Thus, his body learned to store whatever he ate (carbohydrate, protein, and fat). All three of these macro-nutrients are stored in the form of fat because the liver can convert protein and carbohydrates to fat when the hormone, insulin, mediates that activity, and render fat back to glucose later when it's needed. In certain circumstances, the body can also convert protein (muscles) to glucose.

So Urk's body did something wonderful. It learned to store energy two ways. First it stored a small amount of *glycogen* – a massive and quick source of energy like the afterburner on a jet fighter, in case a cave bear jumped up and wanted him for a meal. Second, on a much larger scale, Urk's body stored energy as fat in case times were lean. The body only stores a small amount of glycogen, but it can store massive amounts of energy in the form of fat. With these two systems, Urk could survive the immediate dangers as well as the long winter when food was scarce.

Why does the body store energy as fat? Fat contains more potential energy (calories) than either protein or carbohydrate so it's an effective storage site. Would you want a room full of pennies, a closet full of dimes, or a hand full of gold? The body in its wisdom chooses gold, which nutritionally, is fat.

Macro-Nutrient	Calories (Energy)
Carbohydrate	4.2 / gram
Protein	4.2 / gram
Fat	9.4 / gram

The Urk Gene Factor

Now this story gets interesting because your and my genetics and body processes learned to survive from Urk, the mighty and sometimes not-so-mighty hunter and gatherer. Having stored some extra energy as fat when times were good, Urk was able to access his stored fat and survive when times were lean. Survival gave him the opportunity to perpetuate the species. Urk survived well and married Cinder Crawford, in a touching ceremony where, afterward, contrary to popular myth, *she* beaned *him* on the head and dragged *him* off, and they exchanged the coveted

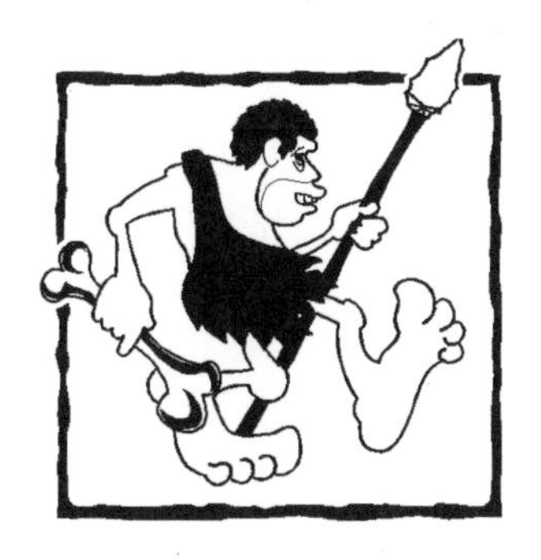

saber tooth tiger-fang necklaces and lived henceforth as family.

Cinder was also a survivor, and, thus, future generations (you and I included) have what is now known as the *enhanced* Urk gene. The Urk gene teaches our body to store energy in the form of fat because the time of famine may come any day. By being such good survivors, Urk and Cinder invented the first yo-yo diet of burning fat through starvation, but then quickly gaining it back when food was eaten.

Our lifestyles are different from Urk's. Through the eating of refined sugars and excessive grains and starches, we not only gain the weight to survive the tough winter; we lock in the fat and make it inaccessible because insulin becomes dominant in our metabolisms. Many people today have huge bank accounts of energy (stored as fat) but the bank is closed and they can't get at it.

Why Calorie Reduction Diets Don't Work

The concept of reducing calories to lose weight is basically a myth. It was perpetuated by the diet industry to justify their programs. It's true that a starving person has low caloric intake and low weight, but, metabolically, the calorie concept is oversimplified, and virtually meaningless. A calorie is a unit of energy. How much energy equals one calorie? It's the energy required to raise the temperature of one cubic centimeter of pure water one degree at sea level.

Many people today base their diets and thus their health on calorie counting charts, not realizing that the charts are inaccurate in the dynamics of nutrition. To calculate calories in a food, a machine burns a speck of food and determines how much heat was produced. Then a caloric value is assigned. However, there are significant flaws in that "scientific" measurement.

- The body does not burn food with fire, but with chemical processes.
- The body does not assimilate the fiber in a food that the machine burned and counted as calories.
- The body does not assimilate the portion of food it does not effectively digest.

Further, calorie-counter people figure that since fat has more calories, it must be fat that makes people fat. Not true. As we'll establish in this chapter, **it's the sugar that makes most people fat**. Eating too much fat, and particularly wrong kinds of fat, can contribute to obesity and other problems, but it's the carbohydrates that take the lead role. In addition, you'll learn later that **you've got to eat beneficial fats to lose fat**.

This process of saving a little for the lean times creates a big problem for people who try to lose weight by cutting way back on their foods and calories today. Not only do they cut back on their nutrition and cause numerous other hardships on their bodies, but also, as soon as they begin eating regularly, their Urk genes start storing fat. This yo-yo effect is heart breaking for obese people because they often think they are to blame or that they are weak-willed. They don't realize it's the perfect expression of their bodies to survive in Urk's hostile environment.

Being adaptable, the Urk gene stores a little more fat than last time, just in case. Thus today, a person restricts calories, loses weight, and eats a pound of food, and gains five pounds back. This system worked great for Urk and Cinder, but for us today, it means that drastically reducing calories is not the way to genuinely lose weight.

Further, during starvation or low-calorie "crash" diets, the body automatically shifts its metabolic processes to a slow, frugal rate. The body instinctively conserves its energy reserves. This is a reason why reducing calories and starvation diets to lose weight don't really work. Besides, it's frustrating to fight yourself.

This chapter will show you how to evaluate how well your body's glucose metabolism is working, so you won't fight yourself. You will see how the process is designed to work, then can answer some self-tests which will give you insight into how well your metabolic processes perform.

How We "Break" Our Metabolic Machinery

Here's how our metabolic machinery is supposed to work. It's a thing of wonder. Our bodies, like the vaudeville plate-spinner, add just enough spin to any plate that begins to wobble to keep it balanced. Most people have heard of the hormone *insulin.* We know that many diabetics need to take shots of insulin to stay alive. Beyond that, not many people understand that insulin is a master hormone that regulates many other body functions, including the storage of fat! Below is a list of insulin's various roles in the body. Notice how many are linked with undesirable effects if overdone. Keep in mind that an elevation of carbohydrates and refined sugars in the diet is what activates insulin and causes its role to dominate.

Insulin:

- Lowers blood glucose levels,
- Provides glucose (and other sugars) for cellular energy,

- Transports amino acids and minerals into the muscle cells,
- Stores carbohydrates (glucose in the blood) as fat,
- Stores serum and lymphatic protein as fat,
- Stores fat (blood lipids) as fat,
- Increases blood cholesterol levels by stimulating the cells to produce cholesterol,
- Causes the kidneys to retain water,
- Increases smooth-muscle-cell growth to thicken artery walls, elevates blood pressure,
- Inhibits the liver's and cells' ability to convert fat to glucose,
- Participates in growth regulation and may cause "activation" of genes associated with obesity,
- Suppresses the immune system by stimulating prostaglandin E2, a micro-hormone that inhibits the effectiveness of the natural killer cells and decreases oxygenation of cells.

The following table is a brief summary of the metabolic pathway that is causing much of the obesity today. This summary illustrates how the body's natural checks and balances to this system can fail when they are overridden or weaken with time and wear out. Today's current eating practices have stressed our systems by over-stimulating them with refined, processed carbohydrates. Eating too many refined carbohydrates has caused insulin to force our cells to accept more glucose than they needed, which has been stored as fat. If this is the case, why isn't everyone fat? The answer is that the body has checks and balances to the runaway effects of insulin.

The primary check and balance to insulin is the hormone glucagon. Basically, it does the opposite of insulin.

Glucagon:

- Elevates low blood sugar,
- Converts protein to glucose, if needed,
- Converts fat to glucose, if needed,
- Activates ketosis, converts fat to ketones for energy, if needed (burns fat),
- Lowers the liver's and individual cells' manufacture of cholesterol,
- Stimulates the kidneys to remove extra water weight,
- Helps the smooth muscles of the arteries relax (lowers blood pressure).

Metabolic Pathway Causing Most of Today's Obesity

A person eats a meal that is high in carbohydrates (starches, sugars) which is quickly digested and absorbed as glucose (pure sugar).

The blood glucose level rises.

The pancreas secretes insulin to deliver the glucose to the cells for energy and to prevent the blood sugar from rising too high and becoming dangerous.

Comment: If the pancreas does its job accurately in dosing insulin, all is well. Further, the presence of glucagon will prevent the blood sugar from dropping too low. Balance is maintained.

If the pancreas secretes too much insulin due to the shock of refined sugars, then the blood sugar drops too low and triggers an alarm response.

Comment: The pancreas must produce glucagon to hold the line for metabolic balance and prevent blood sugar from dropping too low. At this point, the system works after exerting a check and balance system.

↓

Having had too much glucose too many times, and supported by the presence of stress hormones, the cells resist the acceptance of glucose. The glucose stays in the bloodstream longer along with insulin.

Comment: The pancreas thinks it is dosing the right amount of insulin. It did not realize that the cells would be stubborn and require a greater push.

↓

Sensing the elevated glucose, the pancreas produces more insulin to force the glucose into the cells to protect the body from elevated glucose in the blood.

Comment: Now the situation is that insulin dominates the metabolism. Over a longer period of time, insulin is controlling the metabolic processes, while the cells gradually surrender to accepting more glucose.

Insulin, when dominating the metabolic processes, causes fat to be stored and inhibits the hormonal activity that burns fat.

Comment: The end result is fat-gain or obesity.

Insulin and Fat-Storage Obesity

Now, you might be wondering where this lesson in glucose metabolism is going. I certainly hope you are enjoying this brief look into how your body works. Let's look a bit more at the impact of this lesson.

Insulin is responsible for much of the world's obesity. Why? Carbohydrates in our diet quickly activate insulin secretion. The pancreas keeps approximately 200 units of insulin stored and ready for work. Generally in a day's activities, the body will need around 25 to 30 units to handle glucose metabolism in today's high-carbohydrate diets, though it was considerably less a hundred years ago. Besides glucose metabolism, insulin also mediates other processes that we are very interested in, primarily, the storage of fat. Remember, insulin is a fat-storing hormone and its weaker counterpart, glucagon, is a fat-burning hormone.

Insulin's role is to help put glucose (sugar), as well as nucleoprotein and fatty acids, into the individual cells for energy and cellular function; and to store any extra macro-nutrients from the diet as fat for future use. When we eat, digestive enzymes convert carbohydrates (fruit, vegetables, bread, soft drinks, potatoes, grains, rice, desserts, etc.) into a sugar called *glucose*. As our blood sugar (glucose) levels rise while eating, insulin is secreted to move it from the bloodstream into the cells where it is needed. This serves two purposes:

- it provides the energy the cells crave and
- it prevents blood sugar from rising to a dangerous, life-threatening level.

What happens when, day after day, we eat an excessive sugar diet that is depleted in true nutritional value? The systems of checks and balances wear away, for some people faster than for others. One truth is inevitable for everyone — eating an excessive sugar diet moves the body toward the full expression of insulin dominance. Some people have genes that make them very susceptible to the effects of insulin. Approximately a third of the population has this sensitivity and are more prone to gain weight in the presence of excessive dietary carbohydrates. Coincidentally, one in three Americans are overweight. Further, people who do not fall into this category can "earn" this category in time through over-stimulation of the glucose metabolism through dietary sugars. This is one reason why generally fit people gain weight when they turn 40

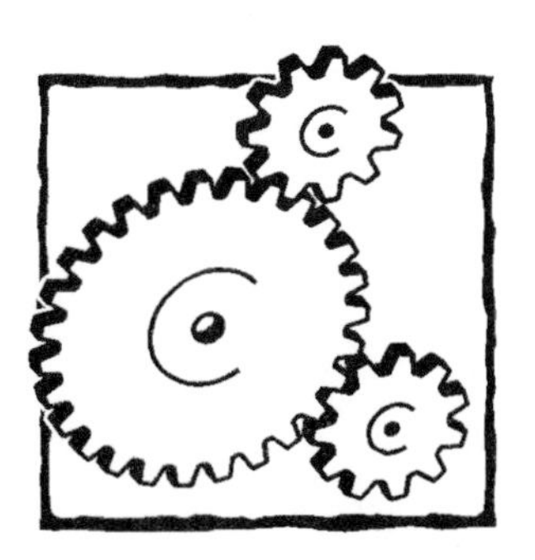

or 50 years old and their metabolic processes naturally shift gears to a slower sprocket.

Although our focus here is on the insulin metabolic pathway, it's important to realize that the body has an intricate system of checks and balances so it can regulate its metabolism and survive. Imbalances in the glucose metabolism can come from several sources, but the one we are focused on here is insulin, and insulin is a hormone primarily controlled by what we eat and how we eat it.

From this one metabolic pathway, there is much more of the story to tell. There are other factors that actually can make the situation worse, and there are factors that make it better. Next, we'll discuss two conditions that can result when this process breaks down, and give you two self-tests to evaluate your risk for both low and high blood sugar conditions. After that, in "The Hormone Merry-Go-Round," we'll continue our investigation of how our metabolic machinery should work and provide a third self-test for another metabolic condition that can make you store fat – insulin resistance.

Hypoglycemia – Low Blood Sugar Condition

Problems with glucose metabolism are often first noticed as a low blood-sugar condition called hypoglycemia, which appears to be the opposite of diabetes, but is really a precursor to diabetes. This syndrome became the "ailment in vogue" in the 1970's, largely due to the rise in refined sugar intake in the American diet. The late 60's and early '70's saw a dramatic rise in the processed, canned, packaged and fast foods that contain hidden sugar and refined carbohydrates.

Hypoglycemia is most often caused by the intake of excessive refined sugar and carbohydrates. Such empty-calorie sugars shock the pancreas into secreting too much insulin. This drives the blood sugar too low. The symptoms of hypoglycemia include irritability, headaches and weakness if a meal is missed, fatigue and sleepiness after eating, and sugar cravings.

Got the high-lows? Too much sugar causes low blood sugar.

Subsequent generations began experiencing hypoglycemia at younger ages coinciding with the rise in refined carbohydrates in the diet. Today, we see hypoglycemia in teenagers because they have been brought up all their lives on sugared breakfast cereals, pancakes, candy, and soft drinks. Is it any wonder that over 25 million people are diabetic in the United States when only 40 years ago there were less than a million? The rapid rise in diabetes far outpaces the increase in population.

Doctors cite "genetics" as what causes hypoglycemia and diabetes. The nutritional perspective is that, "Yes, indeed, millions of people have genetics that make them sensitive to insulin problems." However, it's the improper diet (predominately the use of post-Industrial Revolution refined sugars and excessive carbohydrates) that makes people "earn" the disease (i.e., push themselves into the manifestation of their genetic tendency). The natural health literature cites numerous and frequent examples of how hypoglycemia and adult-onset diabetes can be stopped and reversed with the proper diet and nutritional supplements.

Hypoglycemia is diagnosed by a medical test known as a Glucose Tolerance Test. The test is rough on people with hypoglycemia because, after fasting, they must drink sugar syrup with artificial food coloring in it to challenge their glucose metabolism. Although the following questionnaire is not conclusive or diagnostic, it is accurate in showing if a person has a tendency toward hypoglycemia.

Hypoglycemia Questionnaire	Y or N
1. Crave sweets	___
2. Anxious edge to personality, nervous	___
3. Sleepy shortly after a meal	___
4. Pulse races after eating sweets	___
5. Vision fades when standing up suddenly, dizziness	___
6. Eating starch or sweets relieves headaches	___
7. Irritable, jittery, shaky, if meal is missed	___
8. Appetite increased, frequently hungry	___
9. Calmer after eating	___
10. High carbohydrate diet (vegetarian, low protein)	___
11. Forgetful, weak memory	___
12. Restless mind, poor concentration	___
13. Hungry 1-3 hours after a meal	___
14. Falls asleep easily if activities stop during day, drowsiness	___
15. Fatigue is a chief complaint	___
16. History of low thyroid	___
17. High stress lifestyle for extended periods (worry a lot)	___
18. Wakes at night to eat	___
19. Desires sweets right after eating	___
20. Heart palpitations after eating sweets	___
21. Needs caffeine to get day underway	___

If you answered 3 or more Yes, there is a possibility that hypoglycemia may be occurring.

It is interesting to note that hypoglycemia can mimic depression. Here is a list of mental and emotional states often associated with depression that are also key indicators of hypoglycemia:

Apathy	Forgetfulness	Moodiness
Appetite loss	Headaches	Nervousness
Crying easily	Heart irregularities	Sadness
Detached, disconnected	Irritability	Speech difficulties
Disorientation	Judgement poor	Suicidal thoughts
Dizziness	Low or absent libido	Vision, Blurred
Exhaustion	Memory poor	Weakness
Fatigue	Mental confusion	Worry, excessive

Hyperglycemia – High Blood Sugar Conditions

Hypoglycemia is the forerunner of Diabetes (**Hyper**glycemia.) It is the first, early warning symptom that the glucose metabolism system is under dietary stress. How fast will a person with hypoglycemia develop diabetes? Factors determining how fast hypoglycemia may develop into hyperglycemia include:

- the rate at which sugars and starches are consumed in the diet (how often the pancreas is shocked with a rush of sugar),
- the rate at which the three other hormones that play a role in glucose metabolism (glucagon, human growth hormone, cortisol) become ineffective or over-dominant,

  and
- a person's genetics.

As the hypoglycemic problem continues over time, the pancreas exhausts itself and cannot produce insulin, blood sugar rises too high and spills out in the urine. There are other reasons for pancreatic failure to secrete insulin, including genetics and viral damage, but, when the pancreas cannot produce insulin, the disease is called sugar diabetes, hyperglycemia, or Type I Diabetes. If the pancreas is producing insulin, but it's not enough to stimulate the cells to receive glucose, then the blood sugar rises too high. This is called Diabetes Type II. Below is a questionnaire to determine if you have a tendency toward the blood sugar rising too high.

Hyperglycemia Questionnaire	Y or N
1. History of diabetes in ancestry	___
2. Night sweats	___
3. Deteriorating eyesight (rapid failing)	___
4. Craves sweets, but no relief after eating them	___
5. Increased thirst	___
6. Cuts and bruises heal slowly	___
7. Frequent infections, simple cuts easily infected	___
8. Weight gain, fat gain, over-weight	___
9. High carbohydrate, low protein diet	___
10. Passes sugar in the urine	___
11. Itchy skin, no apparent cause	___
12. Leg sores, boils, skin eruptions	___
13. Fatigue is an ongoing concern	___
14. Mental confusion	___
15. Better energy after exercise	___

If you answered 4 or more Yes, elevated blood sugar may be a concern.

Insulin has a partner in regulating blood sugar. It's the pancreatic hormone, glucagon, which prevents the blood sugar from falling too low after insulin is secreted. Thus, insulin is the hormone that prevents hyperglycemia (elevated blood sugar), and glucagon is the hormone that prevents hypoglycemia (low blood sugar). Together, they make a team of checks and balances so the blood sugar is maintained in the range that supports life. *Too much or too little blood sugar results in death, so the body takes the job of maintaining correct levels of blood glucose very seriously.*

During times of starvation, fasting (controlled starvation for rejuvenation purposes), and excessive physical exercise, glucagon helps the body access its fat-stores and protein (amino acid) structures in the muscles and other organs so the liver can convert them to glucose to prevent death. During such a time of starvation or cleansing, the body literally feeds on itself to maintain its metabolic functions.

The key to life and the key to nutrition is balance in all things.

Here we have a very important principle of nutrition – balance. We encounter this over and over again. Too much or too little creates a problem. This applies to food, vitamins, exercise, antioxidant nutrients, hormones, and life in general, yet we so often see it neglected with people who overeat or take too many vitamins. Glucose metabolism is a balanced system. Two primary and two secondary hormones, plus other factors, work in conjunction with or in opposition to each other to control this essential system. Our lifestyles put stress on this system in several ways. Under stress, this system functions in its default mode for safety and survival. The default is weight gain through the storage of fat.

The Hormone Merry-Go-Round

Just so you'll know there are some other elements to our single-focused story about glucose and insulin, let's take a brief look at some of the other players that affect how the body stores or burns fat.

The table below summarizes these hormones and their function.

Hormone	Gland	Function re: fat storage
Insulin	Pancreas	Lowers blood sugar, stores fat
Glucagon	Pancreas	Raises blood sugar, burns fat
Somatostatin	Pancreas	Bolsters digestive enzymes
Cortisol	Adrenals	Anti-inflammatory steroid, insulin resistance
Human Growth Hormone (HGH)	Pituitary	Converts fat to muscle during sleep if no insulin present in blood

From its location in the middle of the abdomen, the pancreas performs vital digestive processes by secreting digestive enzymes to process all three macro-nutrients – protein, carbohydrates and fat. In addition to the pancreas' vital digestive functions, as we have already discussed, it serves as an endocrine gland in that it puts hormones directly into the blood stream. In this capacity, the pancreas's beta cells secrete the hormones *insulin* and *glucagon*, as well as *somatostatin*, a hormone that bolsters the digestive enzymes. Insulin and glucagon regulate glucose metabolism to maintain proper blood sugar. Insulin is concerned with the storage of fat, and glucagon can help the body access those fat stores to burn for energy.

Two other hormones have a relationship with insulin and glucose metabolism as they work for overall metabolic balance and handle special situations.

- Among many other duties, *Human growth hormone* (HGH) from the pituitary gland works to convert fat to muscle for body repair processes *when insulin is not present in the blood.*
- Among other duties, *Cortisol* from the adrenal glands helps maintain glucose in the blood during times of great stress. It can cause the cells to be more resistant to the effect of insulin to push glucose into the cells.

Have you ever been forced to do something you did not want to do? If so, you probably resisted in some fashion. Imagine that you are being force-fed after you already had enough to eat. If someone actually pried open your mouth and tried to stuff more food in, you might turn your head, spit, bite, kick, and push away. That's what can happen with your cells when insulin keeps forcing dietary glucose into them. They resist because they need to retain their own integrity. This state is called "insulin resistance." Insulin resistance is a problem because it makes the pancreas secrete even more insulin to do its job.

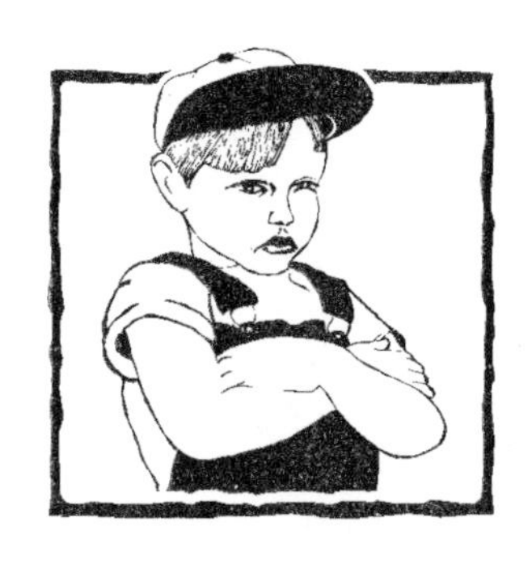

During sleep, the pituitary hormone called *human growth hormone* is released and causes fat to burn and lean muscle mass to increase. This is the body's repair mechanism at work. It's a wonderful ally both to weight loss and optimal health as long as insulin doesn't shut it down. *The secret to increasing human growth hormone production is exercise.*

The adrenal hormone *cortisol* plays a role in glucose metabolism that can cause it to be an enemy to weight loss. It can inhibit weight loss by causing a cellular resistance to insulin and increasing body fat. What brings on the cortisol to foil our plans of rapid weight loss? The answer is stress.

Do you have any big stresses in your life that cause a constant state of worry? Problems at work, problems at home? If you live in a perpetual state of stress, then your stress hormone, *cortisol*, is probably elevated. Further, coffee drinking contributes to the overproduction of cortisol, so people who need a cup or three of coffee to kick off the day are prone to insulin resistance.

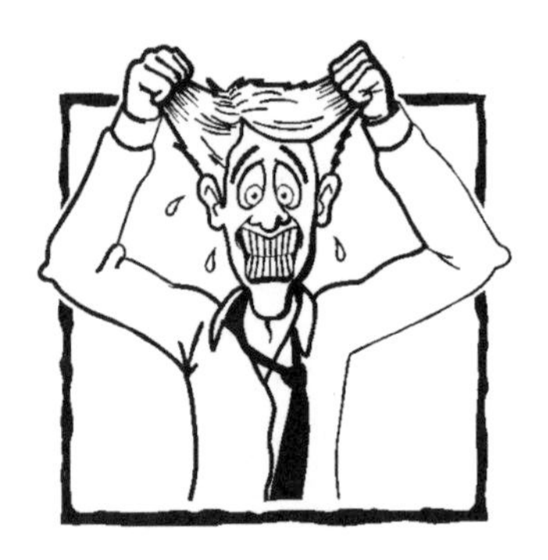

During a time of stress, the body recognizes that its survival is at stake. Stress causes a "flight-or-fight" response and immediate energy (blood sugar) is instantly required when we perceive stress. This life-saving fuel is channeled away from ordinary endeavors and is ready for the muscles to grab and run. This is the self-preservation mode. Since death from a "stressor" may occur much faster than death from starvation, cortisol steps in and claims some authority over glucose and maintains blood sugar to make it available to the muscles for flight or fight responses. Cortisol, an adrenal gland hormone also known *as hydrocortisone*, supports the cells in resisting glucose. With cellular resistance to insulin, the pancreas's tendency is to elevate insulin. This is part of the complex checks and balances, and "domino effect" that hormones cause.

For most people today, the bear doesn't jump out of the cave and end the stress when we run away or fight. Instead, the stress goes on and on. This is the basis of the phrase "adrenal burn out." If your diet is delivering too much glucose, the pancreas must respond by releasing insulin, but the cells say, "Stop, I've had enough," especially if we are under stress, and, frankly, who isn't?

When the cells resist insulin and refuse to cooperate, the excess glucose is stored as fat. So here comes the fat-weight gain and obesity issue. In the short term, excess glucose is stored as fat. In the long term, insulin resistance can develop into Adult-Onset Diabetes. If the insulin-resistant situation continues, the body maintains an abnormal level of insulin in the blood. Even a little bit of insulin stops the body's ability to access fat for energy. The *carbohydrates* in the diet (that keep the insulin levels elevated, the fat increasing and locked in) are the nemesis of people who need and want to lose fat and lower their weight.

Think about it. When does your body have periods of time without insulin dominating the hormonal processes? Do you eat sugar all day in the form of potatoes, cereals, pasta, breads, candies and soft drinks? What about the ice cream or cracker snack before bed? The insulin needed to handle these foods blocks your ability to burn fat via glucagon and human growth hormone. Some people have elevated insulin levels all the time. They never get a chance to lose weight, because of what and when they eat.

Now you can see why some people have had good success losing weight with a high protein diet. Dr. Atkins is famous for this approach and has helped many people who need a drastic, supervised approach. Without the carbohydrates locking in the fat, and with protein's ability to bring forth the fat burning hormone, glucagon, as well as HGH, people experience the conversion of fat to cellular fuel and burn weight away.

There are drawbacks to a high protein, low calorie, low carbohydrate, low fat diet.

- Ketosis (a starvation mechanism where the body shifts its energy source from carbohydrate to fat) can inhibit glucagon.
- Muscle loss can occur.

- Further, the Urk gene can plot to restore the fat as soon as it can. With some people, the protein will stimulate insulin release and block their efforts.

These are some of the reasons a high protein crash program is best attempted in a monitored environment.

The biggest secrets are often discovered right under our noses. The secret to fat burning is simply balance. Balance is something we actively do, not just something we avoid.

Ultimately, all roads lead to the Rome of a balanced diet, and a balanced diet is an individual determination. It is the safe and sensible way to shift weight to the right side of the equation. The secret to burning fat is simple – take the balanced diet and tip it slightly to the fat-burning mode. Modifying your diet to accelerate your fat-loss, within safe and effective parameters, is why the FitTest is important.

What is your level of insulin resistance? Are you eating too many carbohydrates and increasing your fat storage beyond what your metabolism can burn? This questionnaire cannot diagnose insulin resistance, which is the domain of a lab test, but it can give you a clue if you are susceptible to developing this dreaded condition. Insulin Resistance is one factor that the FitTest investigates.

Predisposing Factors In Insulin Resistance	**Y or N**
1. Elevated glucose, when fasting (above 110)	___
2. Had diabetes during pregnancy (gestational diabetes)	___
3. History of hypoglycemia (low blood sugar)	___
4. Poor glucose tolerance (during lab test)	___

5. Adult onset diabetes (Type 2) ___
6. Elevated blood pressure ___
7. Elevated triglycerides ___
8. Ovarian cysts (polycystic ovaries) ___
9. Ancestors had diabetes ___
10. Ancestors had elevated blood pressure ___
11. Ancestors had elevated triglycerides ___
12. Family history of heart disease ___
13. Elevated uric acid (>7.9 on blood test) ___
14. Diagnoses of heart disease ___
15. Sedentary lifestyle, absence of aerobic exercise ___
16. Premature birth ___
17. Birth weight under 5.5 lbs. ___
18. Weight gain > 20 lbs. since age 18 (women), age 20 (men) ___
19. Weight about the same, but fat percentage increase ___
20. Waist over 30" (women), 36" (men) ___
21. Ethnic groups who have adopted a "Western" diet. ___

    Ex: American Indian, Naruans, Aborigines, Maoris, Hawaiians, Polynesians, Melanesians, Hispanics, Japanese, Africans, etc.

22. Craving for sugars and breads ___

22. Elevated cholesterol ___

23. Need coffee to start the day ___

If you scored more than 5 yes answers, you may be experiencing insulin resistance. The degree of insulin resistance can be determined by a lab test.

Four Lifestyles That Help You "Earn" Insulin Resistance

There are other ways to earn insulin resistance other than by eating sugar or having a genetic predisposition to it.

Lifestyle 1: Skipping breakfast

This is a big one. During sleep, the body's metabolism has continued to work. In fact, your body burns a majority of its calories during sleep. The muscles burn fat and glucose. On waking, the body's reserves are low. It's time to break the fast. With the activities of the day, more energy is expended. As blood sugar drops lower with the morning's activities, the pancreas becomes more and more ready to drive glucose into the starving cells. Like a track runner before the starting gun, the pancreas is ready to do its job. This causes the over-exuberance that will slowly develop insulin resistance over time as the body is forced to adjust to a more rapid pushing of glucose into the cells. Even a tiny, balanced breakfast served on a saucer or a properly balanced food bar can prime the fat-burning hormone "pump" through blood sugar stability. Thus, breakfast is essential for the dietary control of the fat-burning mechanism.

Lifestyle 2: The Humongous Supper

Eating lightly all day and then overeating at supper is another way to earn insulin resistance. Dieters often do this. They start the day with good intentions and eat lightly. In the name of calorie reduction, they skip lunch. But by supper, their bodies are screaming for the comfort and well being of eating. So, having been so "good" all day, the evening meal runs berserk. The person can't shut off the appetite that starts screaming for carbohydrates and emotional gratification.

Oftentimes these people are very dedicated workers. They have a piece of fruit in the car on the way to work and a quick, light lunch eaten while working. Then, after 10 or 12 hours of working hard, they eat a big supper to unwind, relax, and catch up. This big evening meal shocks the pancreas with work, both digestively and with blood sugar control. Further, this is very poor timing. The body is given its primary energy fuel at a time the person is preparing to rest and sleep. The cells know the circadian rhythms and are preparing for rest and repair during sleep. Then a huge load of glucose hits, followed by a huge dose of insulin.

The pancreas gets stretched like a rubber band: too much blood sugar, too little, too much, too little. Finally, it becomes exhausted. This situation becomes more complicated when human growth hormone naturally diminishes with age, the metabolism slows down, and the adrenal glands are on a "hair trigger" to release cortisol due to caffeine intake and the stress of daily life. These lifestyle factors take their toll. We must learn a new lifestyle to break this detrimental cycle.

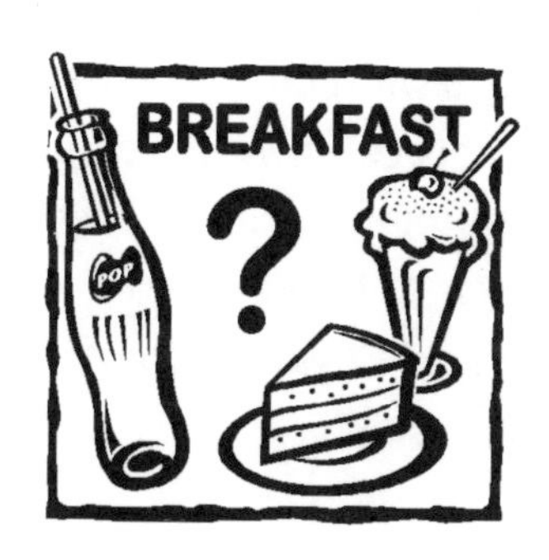

Lifestyle 3: Dessert For Breakfast

A third way to earn insulin resistance is to begin your day with a soft drink or sugared breakfast cereal, or just toast. Pancakes with syrup will do nicely. These sugary/starchy foods convert to glucose at an alarming rate, putting the pancreas into the Rapid Rate Induction Mode. This high/low stretching of glucose metabolism leads to pancreatic overreactiveness which, in turn, leads to resistance of the cells.

Understanding this, we could say that each person has a certain number of "shocks" their pancreas can withstand. Some people can tolerate only a few. These are the obese children, genetically prone to glucose intolerance. Some people can handle

20,000 shocks, so they become hypoglycemic in their mid 20's, and diabetic in their 30's. Other people can take 50,000 shocks and don't have problems until they are in later middle age. Then they blimp out. Finally, some people just seem to get away with it. These are the thin, trim people, who probably smoke and eat all the sugary desserts they want in their late 90's and can't understand what all the fuss is about. George Burns was the "poster child" for this genetic profile with his cigar and martini at age 100. The key element here is: how many shocks can you take? Fortunately, you can get a preview with the FitTest and perhaps get an early warning before serious concerns arise.

Lifestyle 4: Concentrated Protein With Concentrated, Refined-Carbohydrate Meals

Generally, the premise of balanced nutrition is to have all three macro-nutrients on the plate with every meal. This is true, **provided** we apply the *Eating Energy 12 Optimal Nutritional Factors* and avoid the protein/carbohydrate combination that can actually cause an elevation in insulin response. We'll not take on the topic of "food combining" here, but I will point out that when a concentrated protein such as meat is eaten with a concentrated, refined carbohydrate such as instant mashed potatoes, high gluten food like bread, or apple pie, the insulin response can be even greater than eating just the carbohydrate. Here is where the case for quality foods is so important.

Hormone-Balancing, Low Glycemic Meals

Omnivore Meal	Vegetarian Meal
Salmon Filet	Miso with Tofu, Sesame Seeds
Garden Salad with Avocado	Garden Salad with Avocado
Vegetable Medley *(Broccoli, Cauliflower, Green Beans)*	Vegetable Medley *(Broccoli, Cauliflower, Green Beans)*

In a terrific, hormone-balancing, low glycemic meal such as the two in the preceding table, we find protein (fish or miso), carbohydrate (salad, vegetables), and fat (avocado), but these meals do not invoke a high insulin response as a meal featuring a concentrated protein and refined or high-gluten carbohydrate. In contrast, the problem with the "hamburger and a coke" meal, or even "pasta and meatballs" meals is that they combine a solid protein with a high glycemic (sugar) food at the same meal. Here also is the undoing of the dessert after the prime rib meal.

Before you pull your hair out in dismay, rest assured there are simple ways to overcome this problem, which is largely due, once again, to the use of refined carbohydrates. When we learn what proportions of macro-nutrients are right for us, we won't be mislead by the government's Food Pyramid that bases human nutrition on the fluff and dough of carbohydrates. We'll establish our own food pyramid that will build health instead of obesity. We'll use quality foods to build and maintain an excellent degree of health and simultaneously resist chronic degenerative diseases

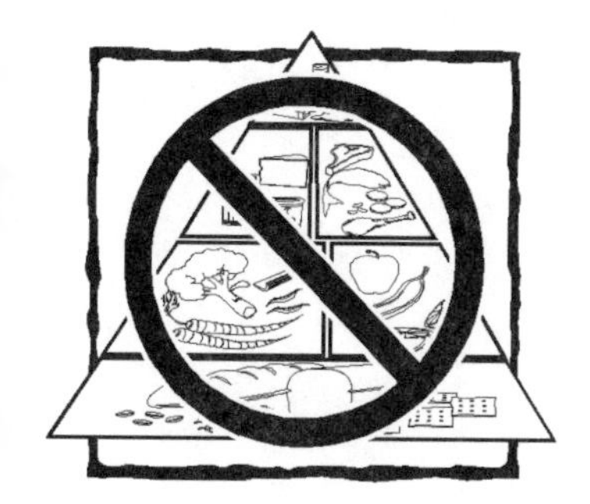

With a little prudence and judgement and some really tasty meals, it's easy to have a totally satisfying meal that supports fat-loss – that's exactly what you'll have with *The Weight Is Over* Program. The next topic may not be suitable for people with delicate sensibilities and a sweet tooth. Parental guidance is recommended – share this information with your children.

CHAPTER FIVE

Sweet Surrender

Nothing is sweeter than the light of truth.
- Cicero

This chapter contains both bad news and good news. First, the bad news – refined sugar sets a trap for your metabolism and can be addictive to both your brain and your body. The good news – you can break these addictions. This chapter's text will tell you how. Read on. Don't give in to a "Sweet Surrender."

In the pre-refined sugar days, from the days of Urk and Cinder to a little more than a hundred years ago, there was very, very little refined sugar in the human diet. The pancreas was used to having glucose enter the bloodstream at a slower, steady pace. For example, in the hunter-gatherer days, the body got glucose from vegetables, which contain fiber, vitamins, enzymes, and minerals. Later, when agriculture became established, glucose came from whole-grain breads, which contained fiber. There is research on Egyptian mummies that strongly suggests that with the founding of agricultural, grain-based communities five-thousand years ago, obesity and heart disease increased dramatically. These cases are cited in the book *Protein Power* by Drs. Eades.

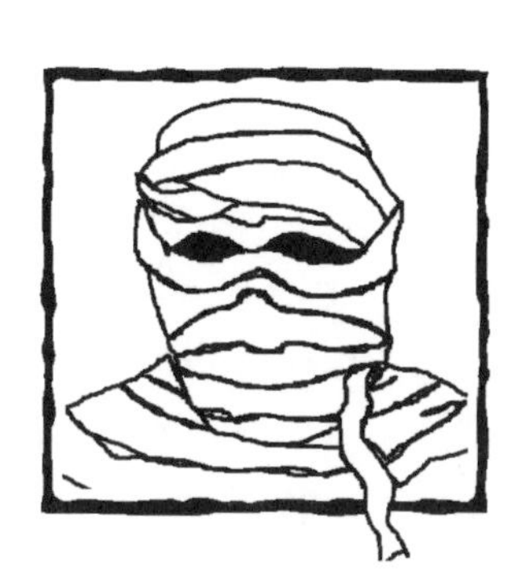

Refined Sugar – The Villain Of The Industrial Revolution

The Industrial Revolution has brought many benefits and an

apparent higher standard of living. However, the Industrial Revolution brought some unwanted side effects. It:

- unintentionally started the process of systematically destroying our health through nutritional depletion, plus
- is a major reason why the United States has such an obesity problem and why juvenile obesity has grown to an alarming state.

Now, enters a new, powerful villain – refined sugar. Coming from the technologies of the industrial revolution, white sugar enters the human diet. In its processed, refined state, it converts quickly to glucose and charges into the bloodstream like a bull in a china shop. Now the pancreas has a powerful adversary, a true challenge.

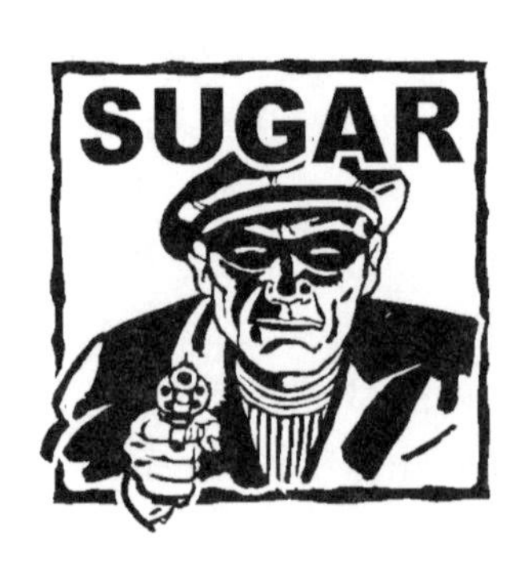

Today, people get glucose from refined sugar with no fiber, no vitamins, no enzymes, and no minerals. There is a big difference, not only in the nutritional value of the foods, but in the rate at which sugar enters the bloodstream. The Industrial Revolution brought the Rapid Rate Induction System to glucose metabolism. The faster sugar gets into the blood stream, the more startled the pancreas is, and the more over-reactive it becomes. An over-reactive pancreas secretes too much insulin. And you know the rest of the story.

How Does Refined Sugar Affect You?

Fabulous research on the effects of the Industrial Revolution's diet of refined sugar and carbohydrate products and cooked foods on indigenous peoples was conducted in the 1930's and published in 1939 by Dr. Weston Price, who traveled the world investigating and documenting the severe decline in health that these foods caused. Dr. Price studied cultures whose diets were based on the local foods. There he found exemplary teeth and no tooth decay, well-formed bones, acute eyesight, and good health. He observed the effects of refined foods on these people as white bread and white sugar were brought into their diets and their health declined. Price kept detailed records and took thousands of photographs. His book, a true nutrition milestone, is entitled *Nutrition and Physical Degeneration.* It is an absolute must for every nutritionist.

Also in the 1930's, Dr. Francis M. Pottenger studied animals, especially cats, to document the decline in health as a result of pasteurizing milk and cooking meat where the heat killed the inherent enzymes and altered Nature's food. He saw gross deformities develop in subsequent generations and extinction by the fourth generation, while the control groups on their natural diet prospered. Basically, Price and Pottenger documented the ancient wisdom at the critical turning point in human nutrition. We still have much to learn from their research.

Now, however, with a single soft drink, a person can have 12 teaspoons of sugar "injected" into their bloodstream with carbonation and phosphoric acid — a genuine threat to balance. The noble pancreas responds with a worthy effort and secretes insulin. Further, many other products from beans to ketchup have "hidden" sugar in them, adding greatly to people's overall consumption of sugar and, thus, to the pancreas's workload. More than that, people do not realize that puffed rice snacks, corn flakes, micro-waved russet potatoes, chips, and white bread pack a sugar punch greater than a spoon of sugar. These "high glycemic" carbohydrates convert quickly to glucose and charge into the bloodstream unchecked, causing an alarmed pancreatic response.

In its exuberance, the pancreas often secretes too much insulin. The cells are force-fed the sugar, the blood sugar drops too low, and the pancreas secretes glucagon to hold the line. The battle is won; the day is saved. Balance is maintained, but the cost is terribly high. Pancreases today are larger and more overworked than they were in the past. People on the post-Industrial Revolution diet have enlarged pancreases. Enlargement of an internal organ is a precursor to disease.

Unfortunately, the soft drink or puffed rice snack is not an isolated instance. Meal after meal, day after day, the refined sugars are poured into the body: sugared breakfast cereals, donuts, sweetened coffee, toast, muffins, croissants, and Danish rolls start the day with a sugar/insulin rush. Then there's the mid-morning soft drink or sugared tea, or pastry. Lunch presents pasta, a roll and piece of pie. Toss in a little candy during the afternoon. Happy hour brings chips and beer. Supper is a baked potato, a roll, a dessert, sweetened coffee. All these foods carry a load of either refined sugar (in the form of sugar) or starch, which the body quickly converts to sugar. The pancreas' silent battle becomes all-out warfare every day.

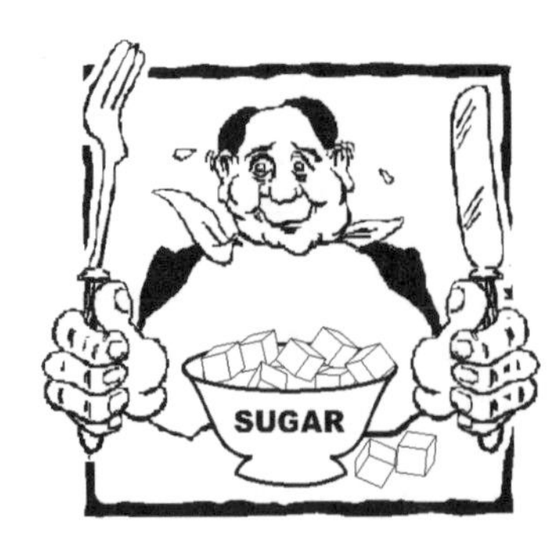

The average consumption of refined sugar, per person, is 146 pounds a year. Adding to that the hidden sugar in the processed foods in the grocery store, the hybridized (sugar-enhanced) wheat and corn that has become a staple food in the USA, a person is likely eating 400 to 600 pounds of sugar a year.

The recipient of all this sugar is the cell. Insulin forces the sugar down the cells' throats because it must maintain proper glucose in the bloodstream. Any excess insulin becomes a problem. Remember that insulin is a fat storage hormone. It also contributes to increased blood pressure, increased cholesterol, increased inflammatory responses in the body, and water retention.

The excessive starches, carbohydrates, refined and processed grains, and "healthy heart" menus all contain high amounts of sugar in the form of refined carbohydrates. Sugar calls out insulin. Insulin stores fat and blocks the burning of fat. Excessive fat is called obesity and presents serious health problems.

Sugar Cravings are Two Addictions In One

Since I have already pointed out the addictive qualities of sugar in a book entitled, *The Next Step to Greater Energy*, (1986) I'll be brief here. Refined sugar is addictive to both

- the body's energy processes and
- the brain's neurotransmitter processes.

Here we're talking about the post-Industrial Revolution processing of cane and beets into empty, white granules called "sugar."

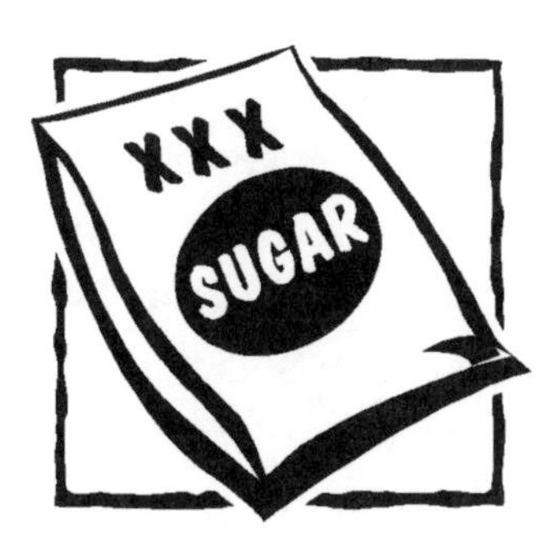

Refined sugar is toxic to the body. It is a poison. It is linked with liver disease, cardiovascular disease, pancreatic disease, cancer, kidney disease, eye disease, dental disease, impotency, hyperactivity, attention deficit disorder, and if you can name it, it's probably linked to or aggravated by sugar. If only people's ears fell off when too much sugar was consumed, the importance of removing sugar from the diet would reach its rightful place of prominence. I hope these revelations about sugar did not come as a shock to you. The nutritional research that shows the detrimental effects of refined sugar goes back many years.

William Dufty presented the case with a nutritional milestone book, *Sugar Blues*, 1976.

It is unfortunate that refined sugar is called a "carbohydrate." This classification dignifies sugar and allows it into the diet. It brings it into the same category as *real* carbohydrate foods such as broccoli and green beans. Poppies are classified as flowers and considered beautiful. Would you allow heroin, the refined, processed, killer drug from the poppy into the "beautiful flower" category?

Sugar Craving Is An Errant Energy-Addiction

Unfortunately, sugar is an area of nutrition people want to ignore. This is because our Urk genes know that having instant fuel is linked to our very core issue – survival. The brain demands glucose – it must have it or die. Many people actually feel better and less depressed, temporarily, after eating sugar. Thus, sugar works its way deep into our bodies, our chemistry, and our psyches.

Better put that cookie back, Mac, it won't build your most precious treasure – your health.

In Urk's day, sweets were roots, tubers, fruit, and honey. The most difficult to acquire was honey, so it was an infrequent sugar experience. Actually, honey is Nature's refined sugar because the bees refine it by predigesting it. The ancient wisdom taught frugal use of honey and the bee taught the price. Fruit in its season provides a sugar called *fructose*. Fructose in raw fruit metabolizes slowly and does not kick the pancreas. Raw fruit is a safe sugar in the natural scheme of things. It is Nature's refreshment.

Urk instinctively sought out sugars. His and our body's "sweet tooth" are actually a survival mechanism in our brains. Unfortunately, we've perverted that mechanism with unnatural foods that tease us with refined, "super-sugar." When our bodies learn there is this really sweet, pure sugar, it causes the "sweet tooth" in the brain to raise its standards. At first, pure sugar was off the chart of experience. Some infants and children naturally reject refined sugar because it is so overpoweringly strong. Over time with frequent exposure, our bodies raise the scale to get refined sugar on the chart. This is the beginning of craving.

Cravings for carbohydrates are often a protein or protein/fat deficiency at the cellular level. Cravings are the body's symptom, a call for balance.

Please understand this. **If you crave sugar, you can overcome that craving.** Sugar craving is actually a protein or protein/fat deficiency at the cellular level. Like the addictive process in the brain involving neurotransmitters and receptor sites, your cells can operate on a high glucose system that constantly needs replenishing. When you stop or greatly reduce refined sweets, your cells will adjust to burning a more sustaining fuel mix, the brain will lower the scale of its "sweet tooth" and you will have peace from the sugar craving.

Here is an example from Ken Robertson of Austin, Texas. This letter came to me while writing this chapter. I found it both timely and appropriate.

> *"As far as diet goes, I've been always at the extremes. Either I was fasting and purifying or living totally on fast foods. Even when I went into my vegetarian mode, I often craved sweets and starches in large quantities and would neglect vegetables and good sources of protein. I've tried all types of eating regimes in the last 30 years. For example, Fruit for Breakfast, while initially very cleansing, it left me feeling weak*

later in the day. Early part of the summer of '99, I was experiencing chronic thirst, blurred vision and frequent urination. I had elevated glucose and triglycerides – classic symptoms of diabetes. I began following the diet in Dr. Tips' book, The Pro-Vita! Plan For Optimal Nutrition, which was on my shelf for years. Here are the results after less than 30 days.

Thirst and frequent urination stopped within 24 hours (which allowed me to get a good night's rest).

More energy, which allowed me the stamina to begin a walking regimen.

Weight loss – I am eating a lot more food (vegetables, low carbohydrate). So far, I've lost 10 pounds in less than a month.

General feeling of well being.

Sharply reduced (90%) my craving for fruit juice and refined carbohydrates like cookies, pasta, and junk food.

I feel as if I am on the right track and that this is not a quick fix but a continued way of living a better life."

Perhaps you have heard, as I have, that, "once a person eats sweets, he or she will want more and more. And if that person quits eating sweets, the desire for sweets diminishes." Thus, eating sweets primes the pump for more sweets. This is really the essence of an addiction. As the body is given more refined carbohydrates and sugars, the metabolic system converts to using more "jet fuel" rather than the body's optimal fuel – a "diesel fuel" of glucose with amino acids and fat. Like a jet fighter that flies at high speeds and whose fuel must be replenished frequently, the body becomes addicted to the quick, high energy of refined sugar. Further, the effect of this detrimental fuel is that more is needed in the wake of its use. This cycle illustrates how the addictive quality of sugar traps the *body's* metabolism.

Sugar Cravings Are A Mood-Altering Addiction

Even beyond the energy aspect, sugar is addictive to the brain. When insulin is produced as a result of eating sugar, many other metabolic processes follow. Insulin allows an amino acid, *tryptophan,* to cross the blood/brain barrier and stimulate the production of a neurotransmitter, *serotonin.* Serotonin fills the beta-endorphin receptors in the brain and, thus, is directly involved with how much happiness and restfulness a person experiences. When serotonin is low in the brain, a person feels depressed, has trouble sleeping, gets headaches, and has a craving for carbohydrates. Many people who are overweight have a bona fide craving for carbohydrates, which is the body's attempt to increase serotonin to feel better. They become addicted to the feeling that sugar gives them.

These people often have elevated monoamine oxidase (MAO), a brain chemical which serves to balance serotonin by destroying it. These people often find that an herb, St John's Wort, can help stabilize the brain chemistry by inhibiting monoamine oxidase, and allowing the presence of serotonin without the sugar craving. However, other substances can fill those receptor sites – morphine, alcohol, and sugar. Thus, excessive glucose can interfere with brain chemistry. It can make a person temporarily happy. But, it is burned quickly in the brain, leaving a deficit or a "sugar blues" that sends a person seeking a carbohydrate or candy. Drs. Phelps and Nourse, in their book, *The Hidden Addiction,* cite sugar as the world's most widespread addiction and perhaps the most hard to kick.

Food is linked with comfort. This began as an infant at the breast. This is the reason many people want to eat sweets when they are sad, frustrated, unfulfilled, stressed, worried, and upset.

"Nothing like a pint of ice cream after a hard day," is a common expression. The sugar provides the comfort and neurotransmitters to help smooth out the rough spots in daily life. Unfortunately, there is a price to pay. This means that another solution needs to be found. Check out gardening, meditation, prayer, reading, learning, exercise, talking, sharing, and frankly, a well balanced meal will fill the bill nicely.

The impact of refined sugar on many people's metabolisms could qualify it as a drug because it dramatically alters body chemistry and can be addictive. It causes changes in behavior and dramatic changes in the body's metabolism, and it has damaging side effects. Yet, a stroll down the aisle in a supermarket reveals large quantities of this substance on children's breakfast cereals, in canned goods, in milk-formula, and in most processed foods. Of course, the manufacturers tell us, "That's O.K. We've fortified the food with eight essential, very common vitamins in synthetic form."

Today, refined sugar would be classified a drug by the FDA if it wasn't already in the public domain.

Unfortunately, it often occurs now that both Mom and Pop work, or that Mom or Pop is a single parent, or that Mom and Pop are too tired, stressed, and overworked to prepare a real meal. After a couple of boxes of dry cereal, the kids are hooked on sugar for breakfast. It is time now to reevaluate our value system. In this book, we learn how to prepare a wholesome, nutritious breakfast. When your children help, breakfast becomes quality time in more ways than one.

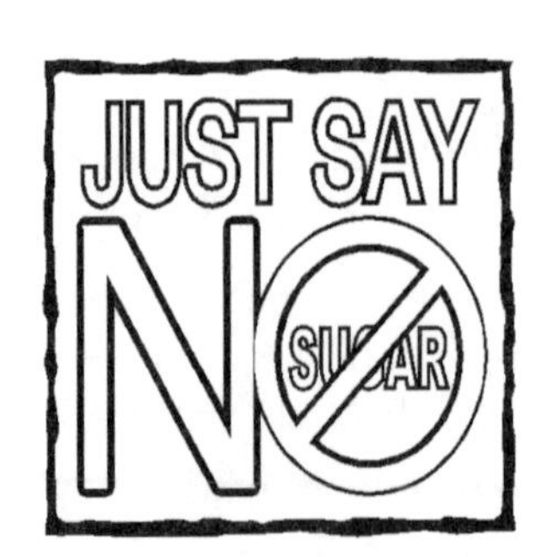

The average American consumes more than 1/3 pound of refined sugar a day! None of this sugar is needed for nutrition. Coincidentally with that rise is also a rise in heart disease and diabetes. Are they related? Many researchers say, "yes." Much of the sugar that people consume is hidden in processed foods – canned goods, baked goods, soft drinks, snacks, desserts. *The best advice is to avoid sugar like the plague it is, then what you inadvertently get will be a manageable amount.*

For sweets, use fruit. You may find that a plate of organic orange sections doesn't last long when the kids are around. The same is true of apple and pear slices, strawberries, pomegranate, and pieces of pineapple. These foods are Nature's true pleasure foods, provide comfort, and are a wonderful after-school snack. The complex and simple sugars can be wholesome, natural foods such as a yam or salad or an apple. Refined sugars are unnatural foods and cause metabolic stress, resulting in tissue damage over time, particularly to the liver and blood vessels.

The Taste Buds And The Refined Taste For Sugar

Why is sugar so addictive? Why does it taste so good? I have a speculation from the ancient wisdom. The human being's sense of taste is divided into four categories. Salt, sour, bitter and sweet. These four categories represent what our bodies choose to taste for survival in a hostile environment.

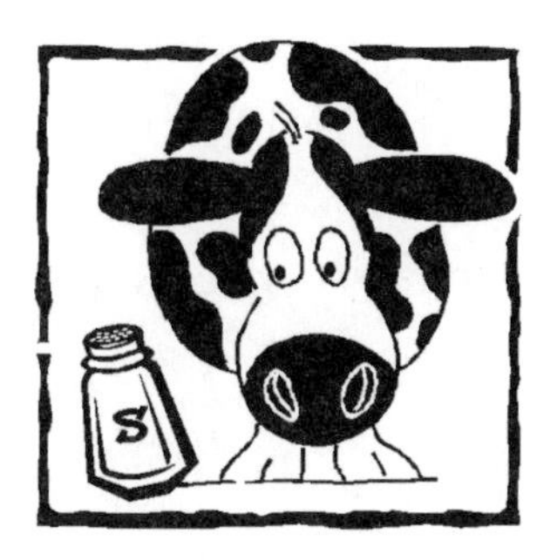

Salt is a need of the body, and mineral salts are vital for health. The best salts come from raw fruit and vegetables, but even sea-salt or rock salt will satisfy the innate, biochemical desire for salt. The tongue locates salt and communicates to the brain that it is available for our biochemical balance. We can desire salt and know it when we taste it. Out here in the cow pastures of Texas, we have something called a salt lick. It's a big block of salt set near the water trough. Oftentimes the cows congregate around the lick to get a dose of salt. They do this instinctively.

Sour is another taste differentiation. It represents another regulator of metabolism such as the citric acids needed for the "food-to-energy" cycles at the cellular level. We can desire sour fruits, vinegar, and tart foods to meet that need for metabolic balance. Sour foods provide certain chemicals that we may or may not need. Some people crave sour foods; some people reject sour foods. At the movie theaters, you'll see a few people who forgo the salty popcorn and the sweet candy in favor of a pickle and maybe some sour candy such as Sour Patch Kids or Lemon Drops. This is the "sour lick" that they instinctively seek.

Bitter is the third taste category. Things that taste bitter usually cause people to avoid them. Many poisonous substances are bitter. So are many medicinal herbs. The bitter taste allows us to differentiate substances that we must avoid or use with prudence and judgement. There are not many people congregated around the "bitter lick."

Finally, **sweet** – the one taste so many desire. The sweet taste results in instant salivation to convert the starches to glucose for immediate fuel. Saliva (containing starch-digesting enzymes amylase and ptyalin) digests only sugars and starches, not other food substances, because the body demands immediate access to its primary fuel and brain food. Glucose is the fuel that keeps us warm in winter and helps us run from tigers. The issue of "sweet" is more closely aligned with immediate survival issues. We have a genetically finely tuned taste for sweet.

In this country, we have set up millions of "sweet licks." They are in our grocery stores, school cafeterias, and movie theaters. They border our roads and highways. They have literally become all pervasive. Coupled with sugar's dual addictive quality, "glucose delivery vehicles" (sodas, junk food, etc.) make the sugar addiction easy to acquire.

With the industrial revolution bringing refined sugar and refined grain products to the world's-plate, our sense of "sweet" becomes warped. Instead of being satisfied with a carrot or piece of fruit, this sweet-sense is stretched or pushed further and further by the constant access to refined sugar. Both taste-wise and metabolically, people become addicted to sugar. Refined sugar has played into our weak link, our body's strong and instinctive desire for energy,

As people break away from their sugar addiction, they often report that they have more energy and better sense of taste and smell. Foods that formerly tasted yucky (such as vegetables) suddenly start tasting good. The removal of excessive sugar also removed the warped or perverted sense of taste and allowed a more accurate sense of taste to develop.

Here is a list of concerns regarding refined sugar, the white granules that are so pervasive in our grocery stores, vending machines, and school lunches.

Sugar Woes

- Refined sugar is addictive. It creates a need to repeat its use.
- Refined sugar is empty calories. It does not provide vitamins, minerals, protein, fatty acids, fiber, water, enzymes, electromagnetic energy or any nutrition to the body as other natural foods do.
- Refined sugar removes valuable nutrients from the body, especially B-vitamins and trace minerals.

- Refined sugar warps our sense of taste and stretches the scale away from nutritious foods in favor of refined sweets and refined carbohydrates.
- Refined sugar is linked with many diseases and disorders.
- Refined sugar creates a metabolism that inhibits the hormone, *leptin,* which turns off the appetite. People who eat sugar frequently often experience an increased appetite. Not good for proper weight!
- Refined sugar creates insulin resistance – a direct pathway to obesity, cardiovascular disease, diabetes, heart disease, and cancer.
- Refined sugar makes people fat.

The Sweet Solution

So, now that we've thoroughly bashed one of the most pervasive, low nutrition food substances in our diets, what's the solution? Fortunately, with some minor changes in lifestyle, excessive use of refined sugar can be avoided. These wholesome and even more tasty solutions will be discussed in the "Substitutions" chapter in Part Three of this book.

Sugar Substitutes – Some Good, Some Bad

Some people think Aspartame or Nutri-Sweet© is a good substitute for sugar. *According to many nutritionists, not so!* This man-made sweetener is linked with mood swings, hyperactivity, attention-deficit disorder, irritability, anxiety, depression, insomnia, headaches, high blood pressure, increased appetite and epileptic seizures. Dr. H.J. Roberts, MD, has published over 500 cases of aspartame-induced illnesses. Aspartame metabolizes into methanol, an alcohol that the body cannot process and finds very difficult to eliminate. Methanol takes five times longer than whisky-alcohol to be eliminated from the body. With these facts, and despite the multi-million dollar campaign to sell the world on aspartame, it is *not* an acceptable substitute for sugar.

Try Stevia as a sugar substitute. It's a natural!

For a quick preview and a ray of hope, the herb, Stevia, from South America, is 200 times sweeter than sugar and it does not contain sugar! It contains an amino acid and, herbally, has a history of helping people with glucose metabolism problems. Many people simply add Stevia to iced tea, pure cranberry juice, coffee, and to baking recipes in lieu of sugar. This can be a valuable transitional factor when people have a strong desire for something sweet because they can deliver sweet to their taste buds without sugar! Stevia is available in health food stores.

Cutting back on sweets right now is a major first step toward good health. Forget the feeble attempt to improve health via "low fat" foods. Low-fat foods generally have more sugar (and less taste) in them than the regular variety and it's refined sugar that's killing people. Natural fat doesn't hurt people; it's the post-industrial revolution processed, partially-hydrogenated fats that are wreaking havoc with our health. We'll tackle some of that issue later, in the chapter on Fats in Part Two.

How far has the sugar/insulin/insulin-resistance issue gone with you? There is now a way to find this out with laboratory testing via the FitTest. Now is the time to initiate positive changes that will affect your immediate and future health.

We've covered a lot of ground and now it's time for a break. Enjoy the next chapter as we go to the feedlot to design some meals for maximum fat gain.

CHAPTER SIX

The American Feedlot – And How To Not

I saw few die of hunger. Of eating, a hundred thousand. - Benjamin Franklin

Are you eating at the feedlot? Sounds unpleasant and uncouth. But let's take a look. In American Agriculture, there is a place called "the feedlot." It's where cows go to fatten up before slaughter. Before going to the feedlot, cows graze in the pasture and eat their natural food – grass. A cow in the pasture will grow up to be lean and rangy. This is their natural state, but lean, rangy meat is not fork-tender, and a lean, rangy cow does not weigh in as high as a fat cow. Thus, a lean, rangy cow will not bring in as much money at market as a fat cow and won't taste as good on the plate. Therefore, ranchers often use supplemental foods to plump up the cows. They also use unnatural growth hormones to help the cows gain weight as fat.

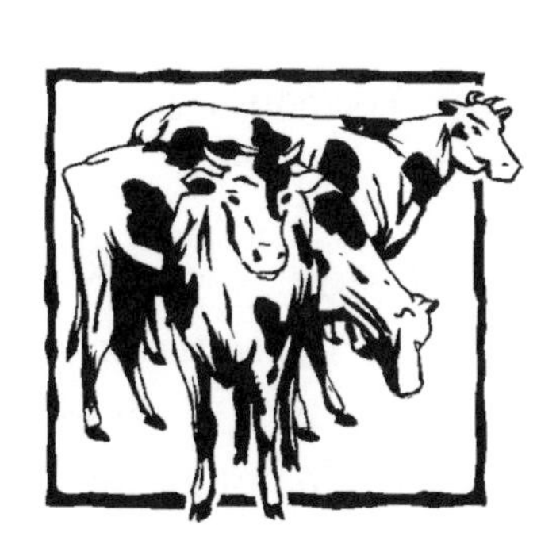

When the cow is ready for market, it goes to the feedlot to add extra fat-pounds before the auction hammer falls. In the feedlot, the cow is force-fed hybridized corn and grains that are higher in sugar than natural grains. Here, the cow becomes fatter. Note: cows *are not fed fat to make them fat, they are fed carbohydrate*. So, from this we learn the law of the feedlot. To get fat, eat a lot of sugar, starches, and carbohydrates, and don't exercise – just like the cow in the feedlot.

Feedlot Meals: Just for fun.

Now, just for fun, let's design some popular feedlot meals. These meals can conveniently be prepared from our grocery stores and health food stores, and are readily found in our restaurants and kitchens.

Feedlot Meal #1-a (Breakfast)

For this meal, let's follow the feedlot principle of using hybridized (sugar-enhanced) grains. The industrial revolution has provided us the technology to create some excellent feedlot carbohydrates: breakfast cereals, microwaved baked potatoes, soft drinks, low-fat milk, and added refined sugars.

Take Nature's corn and hybridize it to make it sweeter, and process it to remove the germ (essential fatty acids), remove the outer layers (minerals, fiber), and create a flake. Now we have a low nutrient, low fiber, high-glycemic carbohydrate. Add a sugar frosting. Let's call this a sugar-frosted corn flake. Serve it in a bowl with low fat milk (which is a high sugar food). The milk is useful also because of the residual growth hormones used to increase milk production in cows.

Serve with a piece of white bread toast. Here the wheat has been processed. The germ has been removed (along with essential fatty acids, minerals, and Vitamin E) and the husk has been removed (minerals, fiber). The flour is bleached to get that "nice" ghost-white color. Char the edges of the bread in a toaster to further break down carbohydrate structures. Serve with jelly or honey to add a sweet flavor and more sugar. To wash it down, a glass of processed orange juice will do nicely. The pasteurization (heating) of the orange juice breaks down the more complex carbohydrates and renders a higher sugar content.

Now we have a meal that meets the feedlot criteria: have dessert for breakfast for maximum fat gain or, if you are young and have not developed insulin resistance, this meal will help you become hypoglycemic, the first step to future diseases.

Feedlot Meal #1-b (Breakfast)

For an alternate feedlot breakfast, let's take the refined wheat flour and make pancakes because the high-glycemic flour converts to glucose very quickly. Add some corn syrup (virtually pure sugar) flavored to taste like maple syrup. Add a little fruit compote to add a festive appearance. Serve with a glass of pasteurized apple juice. To really put the icing on the cake, so to speak, spray on some of that synthetic whipped cream product to add an extra dose of sugar along with micro-fat molecules for instant absorption. We've created a high sugar, low nutrient meal that can cause a sharp spike in insulin and lock in some good fat gain. If this is too much trouble, just make do with cinnamon toast, a bagel, or a donut.

Feedlot Meal #2-a (Lunch)

Spaghetti sounds good. We'll use the refined wheat noodles served in a "healthy heart" marinara sauce made from tomatoes and a "little" sugar. First, include a few bread sticks or a dinner roll. Accompany this with a grated carrot/raisin salad, soft drink and a small piece of cake for dessert. We've successfully created a high sugar meal that can keep insulin pumping!

Feedlot Meal #2-b (Lunch)

Let go to the "vegetarian, healthy heart" menu again and *go a la carte.* Choose the cold pasta salad of curly wheat noodles with garbanzo beans, refried beans with tortilla chips, and corn bread. Accompany this with ice tea with 3 tsp. sugar added, and a piece of bread. It's tempting, so go ahead and add the apple pie. This'll be a killer, high carbohydrate, low fat, low protein meal.

Feedlot Meal #3-a (Supper)

We really should watch our fat intake right? Let's go with a microwave-cooked "baked" potato (97% starch that converts quickly to glucose), with a little margarine. Add a serving of steamed carrots. With it, we'll have a cling peach salad (in heavy syrup.) Might as well have a small portion of sorbet after this high carbohydrate meal. Insulin will have a field day!

Feedlot Meal #3-b (Supper)

Rice sounds good. Let's fix a big plate of instant rice and add some steamed vegetables including carrots, beets, corn, and parsnips. Some corn chips will go great with this. For a drink, cranberry juice cocktail. For dessert, to compliment this natural meal, let's have tofu ice cream.

Any of these meals sound familiar? The criterion used in designing these meals was simply to choose high glycemic carbohydrates. These are foods that quickly convert to glucose and, if unchecked by protein, fat, or fiber in the meal, will cause an insulin rush. With the help from the processing and heating of foods, the nutrition value is lowered and the sugar values rise. This is an excellent scenario for stressing the pancreas and body hormonal balance. Over time, these types of meals will contribute to obesity.

In the Appendix, when we discuss the "glycemic index" of foods (which compares a food's sugar impact as compared to pure glucose) you'll see why these "fun" scenarios pack a wallop of glucose into the bloodstream. We'll learn how to balance a meal to fit our unique metabolic processes and avoid all these problems.

The Role Of Balanced Diets in Healthy Metabolism

In 1995, researcher Dr. Barry Sears authored a pioneering book entitled, *The Zone.* In it, he popularized the role that insulin plays in unleashing a chain reaction of micro-hormones called eicosanoids, which, in turn, control our vital functions such as fat storage, fat burning, how much energy we have, and how well our immune systems perform. He also elevated the role of essential fatty acids in the public's nutritional awareness. In 1996, also from the same perspective, Drs. Michael and Mary Dan Eades authored a book, *Protein Power* that stressed the need to retreat from the high carbohydrate diet. Their success in treating diabetics showed

- the power of a balanced diet over insulin/glucagon metabolism, and
- how glucose metabolism, in the presence of sufficient, balanced essential fatty acids, had power over several critical body processes, including fat gain/loss, the immune system, heart disease and blood pressure.

This research explained the metabolic intricacies of why the book *The Pro-Vita! Plan for Optimal Nutrition* (Tips, 1988) was so effective in helping people lose weight, as well as experience significant health improvements, especially with their immune systems. The Sear's/Eades' research brought to the public eye the complex processes of insulin and essential fatty acids, and showed how a diet of better proportions of macro-nutrients is a powerful tool for health.

The Pro-Vita! Plan established nutritional parameters that challenged the then and unfortunately now-popular high carbohydrate diet and brought an element of metabolic balance through a more healthful approach to eating. Beyond the better balance of macro-nutrients, *The Pro-Vita! Plan* delved into the high-quality vs. poor-quality foods and the importance of all the other nutritional elements such as micro-nutrients, alkaline reserve, electromagnetic potentials of foods, and enzymes.

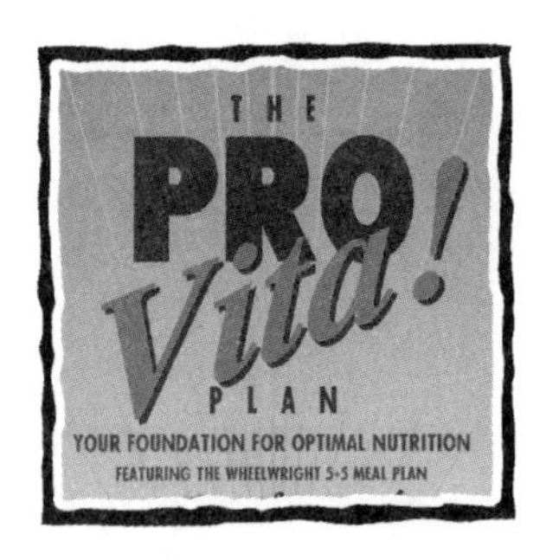

The Weight Is Over nutritional discussion is based on *The Pro-Vita! Plan For Optimal Nutrition,* and provides you the streamlined, essential insights of over 30 years of nutrition research, focused in a way that you will be able to benefit immediately. This means that you'll get the best of macro-nutrient-balance **and** the best of nutritional "ancient wisdom" insights, combined into the most dynamic eating plan of the 20th century. What a great way to launch the new millennium with a complete approach to the best of health!

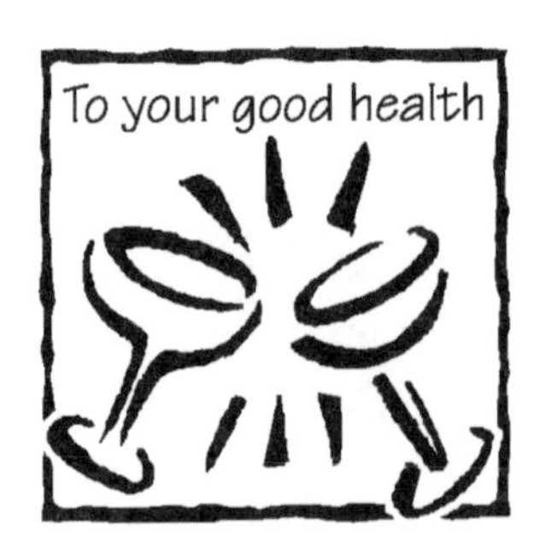

Since the three pioneering books mentioned above, there are a host of other books that now stress the importance of balancing the ratios of the three macro-nutrients. It's the direction in which Nutrition is currently heading. However, to date, none of the other books show the difference between the *quality* of the foods in each category. They attempt to show us how, mathematically, if we have a protein and fat-rich pork chop, we can have a hand full of M&M's candy for the carbohydrate portion and it all balances out to be a meal with favorably ratios. Such a meal can be balanced regarding macro-nutrients, but there are other factors we must address if true health is to be ours. We take all those important factors into account in *The Weight Is Over* Program!

Current programs make an oversimplification that can risk your health. A healthy diet and staying healthy is more than simply balancing carbohydrate intake with protein and fat. A balanced ratio of macro-nutrients is more complex than a one-size-fits-all formula. Fortunately, we won't have to go into a lot of scientific detail to capture the essence and the results of what insulin regulation means to our ability to lose weight. Based on the additional insights of quality vs. quantity, we'll be able to pick the best of the best for an excellent degree of health.

Please remember, this book is for everyone. For the more curious, the scientific side is easily accessible via the bibliography of the book, *Eating Energy*. The chapters in Part Two of *The Weight Is Over* will help you make dramatic changes in your weight and health; and most importantly, you'll learn exactly what to do to protect yourself and your family from the ill effects of an unbalanced diet. Now that we've had some fun at the feed lot and looked at the most current research on diet, let's look at how many diet plans might tell you to eat to burn fat, and compare that to the *Eating Energy* approach featured here in *The Weight Is Over*.

Fat-Burning Breakfast Comparison

Here are two meals that meet the macro-nutrient ratio to allow the body to access its fat stores for energy. The first one (Breakfast A) is a typical, low-nutrient approach. The second one (Breakfast B) is truly enriching. We'll use some of the same foods and demonstrate how a ShiftRight in quality can greatly enhance your nutritional intake.

Breakfast A: Typical, low-nutrient, but macro-nutrient balanced meal

- One raisin or blueberry bagel (approx. 2.7 oz)
- Low fat cream cheese (approx. 1.6 oz)
- Smoked salmon or lox (approx. 3.2 oz)
- Capers (8, not nutritionally significant)
- Orange juice (small, 4 oz.)

Let's look at the components:

Carbohydrate comes from the bagel and orange juice and provides 41.5% of the calories. *Protein* comes from the cream cheese and salmon and makes up 32% of the calories. *Fat* comes from the salmon and a little from the cream cheese and makes up 26.5% of the calories.

So what's lacking? You can figure it out. Just compare it with *the 12 Eating Energy Optimal Nutrition Factors.* Where are the vitamins, minerals, trace minerals, and fiber? Where is its digestive potential and life-factors? I know what some of you will say. "But the orange juice has Vitamin C." And the nutritionist replies, "Well, hoop-tee-doo. Added vitamin C does not a nutritious meal make!"

Now, let's upgrade this meal by our **ShiftRight** technique.

Breakfast B. An Eating Energy breakfast designed for its fat-burning potential and wealth of nutrition for optimal health.

Let's shift the sugar enriched, processed grain, nutrient-depleted, insulin-inducing bagel right off the plate and into the trash. Do not give it to your dog. Instead let's begin with a light and fresh garden salad with a variety of lettuces and crisp vegetables. Here we go!

- Garden salad (2 cups) organically-grown romaine, endive, beet leaf, dandelion, etc., often purchased as a field green mix at the store. Add some sunflower spouts.
- Salad dressing (homemade with olive oil, grapeseed oil, flax oil, lemon juice, ginger and fresh rosemary, kelp, and basil. (2 Tbsp.)
- Salad garnishes: sunflower seeds, walnut pieces, feta cheese, and in a moment of swashbuckling daring-do, go ahead and toss on a couple of croutons.
- Small piece of grilled salmon. (3.5 oz)
- Capers (8, not nutritionally significant)

Now let's look at the components:

- The salad and croutons provide *carbohydrates.*
- The salmon, sunflower seeds, walnuts, sunflower sprouts, and feta cheese provide *protein.*
- The salmon, feta cheese, sunflower seeds, olive oil, grapeseed oil, flaxseed oil, and walnuts provide beneficial *fat.*

Now apply the *Eating Energy 12 Optimal Nutrition Factors.* Holy Cow! We have a nutritional powerhouse of proteins (both raw and lightly cooked) that include a tremendous array of amino acids and a strong showing of complete amino acids. The fats presented actually can help prime the fat-burning mechanism and include Omega 9, 6, and 3 fats and essential fats, as well as EPA and DHA that have been shown to prevent cardiovascular disease. The carbohydrates do something here that no piece of dough can: They provide nascent vitamins, minerals, trace minerals, small amounts of amino acids, enzymes, small amounts of essential fats, water, fiber, and bio-energetic life factors not found in a cooked or dead meal.

Longevity Tip: Life begets life. Have raw, live vegetables with every meal.

With this meal, you have virtually quadrupled the nutritional value and provided missing elements your body craves. Actually, this one meal contains more vital nutrition than many people get into their bodies in a week!

Imagine what this can do for your health when you generously provide your body the raw materials for its vital life processes such as energy, fighting cancer, repairing weak tissue, burning fat, neuro-transmitter balance, and protecting your bones. What a difference it makes!

Now, you're probably saying that the more favorable meal looks a lot like lunch or supper, not breakfast! I can't help that, but I do understand. So if this idea is too radical for you, you'll need to compromise. Instead of a radical ShiftRight, just a little one will do nicely and still make a big difference. A simple way to increase your nutrition without becoming a health nut is simply to have raw vegetables with every meal. This means that you might add a couple of stalks of celery or a small salad with Breakfast A and use only half of the bagel. Then you'll be on the right track. Also, the addition of super foods or supplements can help as well. For instance, adding a green drink or greens in a capsule will provide many of the missing factors.

Have you had a salad, a piece of celery, an apple, an olive, some almonds today? The "back to nature" movement is really a return to basic foods that form the foundation of our health.

So, here's the big question. Do you want to lose fat and still be unhealthy and nutrient-depleted like the multitude of weight loss plans recommend? Or do you want to take a shot at the truly dynamic life you can have with optimal nutritional health? In your hands is a book that truly gives you the opportunity to optimize *both* weight and health. More than a plan, this is a gift. As I write this, I am already looking forward to meeting those of you who will join the thousands of people who take the FitTest and ShiftRight to a more natural diet and set a new standard of nutritional health in their lives.

Optimal Health

Optimal health is our birthright. Our bodies were made to function in good health and vitality. What is the actual state of optimal health? It is much more than "wellness," which is only "the absence of disease." Optimal health is a dynamic, vital state of being where everything works right and we live in a state of peak adaptability and performance.

To me, "absence of disease" means that we aren't getting sick. We are not developing chronic, degenerative diseases. This is a side effect of optimal health, but not the true goal. "Wellness," means not being sick, in body, emotions, and mind. This, too, is only a side effect of optimal health. Imagine what optimal health is like. Feel the magic and ecstasy of good energy, mental clarity, strength and stamina. Feel the self-confidence, inner strength, and heart-centeredness that impart a passion to your daily events. It's OK if you'd like to shout out, like singer James Brown, "Oooooooo, I feeeel good! Duh-da-duh-da-duh-da-duh, I knew that I would!"

Optimal health is the most vital state in which a person can be. It differs from person to person, but there are some common expressions for everyone. A popular example of optimal health can be seen in the public figure Anthony Robbins. When he speaks, you feel his energy, passion, and vitality. It literally crackles around him. When he moves, you see his body is fit and powerful. When challenged, you see he has a good degree of mastery over his emotions that gives him the strength of self-control. When he performs, you see his mind is clear and focused. Thus, his body, emotions, mind, and spirit are in harmony with his purpose. This allows him the joy of minimal resistance and maximal effectiveness in his life endeavors.

Now I don't believe in putting human beings on pedestals, so I'll tell you now that I'm not idolizing Tony Robbins, or anyone else, for that matter. I'm just pointing out a popular, public figure who has dedicated his life to optimal expression of human potential in his chosen arena of human motivation and mastery of life. He exemplifies an optimal life that is right for him. What is the optimal life for you? More energy, less fat-weight, sharper mind, more stable emotions, more financial freedom, more love? We all have a ways to go to unfold the best that we can be.

NATURAL LAW: Adapt or die. Nutrition is fundamental to adaptability.

Optimal health in the physical body is an unobstructed vitality to serve and protect our health.

- It is *a balanced biochemistry* so all the "wheels-within-wheels" activities of hormones and tissue responses run like clockwork. The plates all spin with great adaptability to life's circumstances.

- Also, optimal health includes *a balanced emotional state*. We can fully experience all joys, all the excitement, all the disappointments and grief that we encounter, and have the ability to move back to a well functioning, healthy outlook, so we can complete our life-purpose.

- On the mental level, optimal health means that *our minds are clear and sharp*. Our memory is good. Our insights and intuitions are accessible for creative problem solving.

- And spiritually, optimal health means that the *assimilation of life's lessons make us wise, more loving, more compassionate, less judgmental, and better able to fulfill our true missions in life.*

With all these lofty thoughts, what's the role of diet in all this? Since there is an undeniable interconnectedness between the physical body, the emotional and mental states, and ability to fulfill a spiritual purpose; a healthy, adaptable, vital, well functioning body is a major contributor to a well-balanced life.

NATURAL LAW: Within each of us is a healing, self-regulatory mechanism programmed to operate our bodies in optimal health.

Our dietary health is our responsibility. It is within our control. If our diet is optimal, it can reward us with a most precious commodity that is so fundamental to the quality of life we crave – energy. Diet is essential for optimal health. Optimal health unleashes the energy within us for us to live truly vital lives.

Unleash Your Innate Vitality

Within each of our bodies is the inherent power to heal ourselves, adapt, and maintain balance in all its functions. It does so according to a blueprint established over thousands of years – our genetic code and structure of our enzyme systems. In natural healing, we refer to the body's instinctive healing mechanism by several names including the "Vitality," "Vital Force," "homeostasis," "balance," "equilibrium," and "regulatory mechanism." Whatever it's called, it is energy and it keeps us alive and running. It's the automatic pilot that holds our survival foremost in its actions and directions.

The *Vitality* is very powerful, very instinctive. It maintains our health according to our optimal blueprint as best it can. If something comes along that is perceived as a threat to our survival, the Vitality can react aggressively, even violently, to help preserve our lives. Thus, coughing, vomiting, diarrhea, cold/flu symptoms, discharges, and fevers are the more aggressive tools the Vitality uses to protect us.

Our bodies can heal themselves – if we get out of the way.

Our bodies make thousands of adjustments every hour, automatically. If you are not experiencing all the benefits of great health, the question is, "What is blocking your Vitality from its full expression?" In Chinese medicine, the question would be, "What is congesting the free flow of your ch'i (life) energy?" For many people, diet is a major handicap to a life of optimal health.

Diet can have one of three impacts on our vitality. It can be negative, neutral, or positive.

The foundation to our full expression as human beings is health – something largely dependent on what and how we eat.

- Negative dietary influences include such things as pesticides in commercial meat and vegetables, chemical additives (preservatives, artificial color, aspartame), alcohol, tobacco, chocolate, coffee, partially-hydrogenated oil, commercial milk products and so forth.
- Neutral impact foods include foods that aren't overtly harmful, but don't have much life in them. Overcooked vegetables is an example.
- Positive impact foods invariably have life force in them such as sprouts, raw fruit and

vegetables. These foods are rich in enzymes, vitamins, minerals, water, electromagnetic force, and fiber. Much of the focus of Part Two of this book is to point you in the direction of the positive foods – to give you the knowledge to empower you to use your diet to improve your health.

I recall a lesson of the Vitality from my military high school days. My Vitality made a dramatic adjustment to preserve the status of my health.

On a field trip to the Florida Keys, I got hold of a huge cigar. The thing was practically bigger than I was. I smoked it that night in Miami and it took me three hours of non-stop puffing to finish it off. As you might suspect, I turned green, vomited violently, felt dizzy, nauseous, and absolutely horrible. So why is this a lesson in vitality? Well, it was my Vitality that came to the rescue with violent vomiting in its effort to rid my body of the toxic, cerebrally disturbing effects of tobacco. The tobacco posed a recognizable threat to my health and my Vitality responded with enthusiasm.

The next day, I boarded a bus for Key West. Even though it was ten hours since I last hung my head over the bowl, when the driver lit up a cigar, my Vitality responded again to even the second-hand smoke from the now sore subject, with the same enthusiasm as the night before. My head was quickly out the window. What a powerful ally the Vitality is!

It's easy and colorful to cite the Vitality's positive adjustments to negative influences, and perhaps humorous if you can delight in my rites of passage. However, keep this in mind: Our Vitality can just as assuredly respond to beneficial influences (such as a Positive Impact Diet™) and lift us up to a fuller expression of our innate vitality. When we stimulate our Vitality with a positive impact diet, we realize more of the traits we desire, such as higher energy, clearer thoughts, and freedom from symptoms. Through the use of the ShiftRight technique, a positive impact diet is attained.

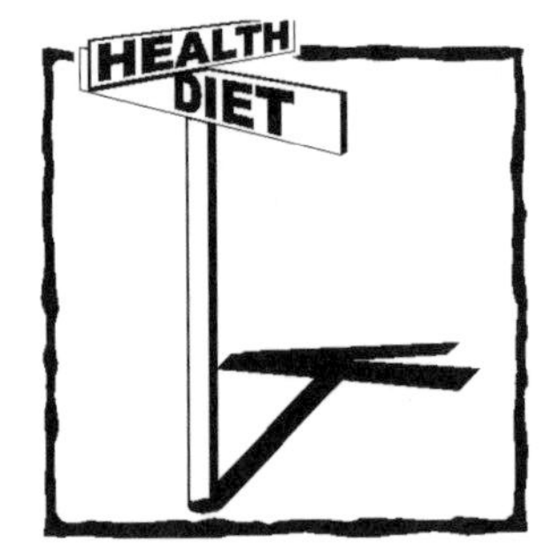

Here we reach an intersection on life's path. It's the crossroads of diet and health.

- Does our diet impact our health negatively and interfere with our innate Vitality, thus contributing to a low quality of health and setting the stage for disease?
- Does our diet impact our health neutrally, being neither too beneficial nor detrimental, letting nature take its course with the aging process?
- Or does our diet impact our health positively and provide the tools the Vitality needs to usher us to optimal health?

Food and Your Internal Terrain

Food is a major contributor to the "terrain" inside our bodies. *Terrain* refers to the quality of our blood and tissues. More specifically, "terrain" refers to the blood and the space between our cells known as the interstitial or intercellular matrix. Our terrain is what either makes us susceptible to diseases by creating a favorable environment for invaders, or protects us from diseases by creating an unfavorable environment for disease-causing agents.

- If our blood and tissues have a lot of toxins and congestion, we have a breeding ground for pathogenic bacteria and virus.
- If our blood and tissues are clean, destructive bacteria and virus do not find a home.

For example, if you want to find the plant known as "cattails," you must look in a sluggish water area such as a swamp or creek, because that is the terrain in which they thrive. Cattails can choke a stream and cause congestion. You will not find them in a rapid flowing mountain stream. In our bodies, if you want to find a breeding ground for pathogenic bacteria, you need to find a terrain where there is toxicity, putrefaction, and congestion. You won't find it where there is purity and circulation.

Why is diet so critical to our internal terrain and, thus, our health? There are several reasons.

1. *Lack of essential nutrients means that the body cannot function well and regulate itself.* This causes deficiency diseases. For example, one little atom of the trace mineral selenium could prevent oxidative damage to a fat molecule in our abdomen. Without that nutrient, the fat oxidizes and sets off a chain reaction that causes a toxic, damaged section of tissue. This weak tissue becomes a breeding ground for a pathogenic form of streptococcus bacteria.

2. *Imbalances in the macro-nutrients (protein, carbohydrate, fats) cause excessive or diminished hormonal responses that result in symptoms* (such as blood sugar imbalances, inflammatory reactions, heart disease and impaired immune response.) These imbalances predispose our health in a negative direction.

3. *Toxins in the food* such as pesticides, growth hormones, antibiotics, partially-hydrogenated oils, and preservatives "trash out" our inner terrain and *must be broken down and eliminated by the liver, or else they block important enzyme activities and alter hormonal responses.*

4. *Some substances used as foods* (refined sugar in soda pop, candy, desserts, etc.) *literally rob vital nutrients from our bodies, leaving a debt that must be paid at the sacrifice of our health.*

5. *Foods support our bodies bio-energetically,* bringing an element of the electro-magnetic "life force" for us to use.

6. *Our access to energy at the cellular level is directed by food.*

7. *Food provides essential nutrients for the maintenance and repair of our tissues.*

Food is a passport to optimal physical health when applied according to the principles of *Eating Energy.*

Food is a powerful factor. Over time, it either makes or breaks our health.

For many people, the terrain is the turning point between health and illness. "Cleanliness is next to Godliness" is an old expression. It doesn't necessarily mean to go scrub the floor and make your bed. It means to keep your body, your "temple," clean so you can be healthy and experience life 100%! Why is that Godliness? Is it just that God is tidy or partial to cleanliness? Or is your internal environment important to your spiritual development and fulfillment of your spiritual mission in life? Food for thought!

Consider this. It's not the cold or flu virus that makes us sick. If our terrain is healthy, the virus will *not* find a suitable home in our bodies and *won't* proliferate. When the terrain is clean, the virus cannot live well there. When our terrain is supportive to virulent activity and proliferation, the virus *will* find a suitable home in our bodies and *will* make us sick. Whether we get the flu or a cold is not solely dependent on the virus; it's primarily dependent on our terrain. Not everyone exposed to the flu gets sick. It's not the virus that causes the miserable cold or flu symptoms, either. It's our Vitality cleansing the terrain via the mucous out the nose, the fever, the swollen glands, the coughing up of mucous.

Poor dietary choices can establish a terrain that stresses both our Vitality's ability to gently maintain optimal health and our immune system. How? We can cause problems by

- eating foods *containing excessive heat-altered proteins* (charred meat);
- eating *excessive, heat-altered saturated fat* (meat fat;) partially hydrogenated and rancid oils (potato chips, shortening, margarine, etc.);
- consuming foods *containing unnatural additives* such as pesticides (sprayed on fruit and vegetables;) artificial preservatives (added to processed foods;) artificial colors;
- consuming *excessive sugar* (candy, soda pop, desserts;) or *excessive starch* (pasta, grains);

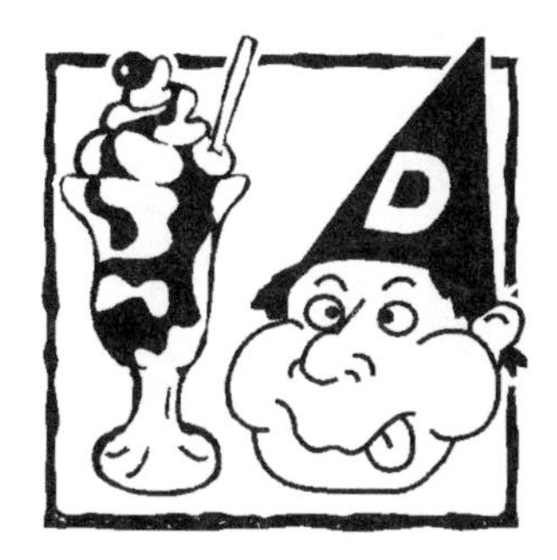

When the body's gentle nudging doesn't work, the Vitality uses stronger methods called "symptoms" to get our attention.

Please note that all three basic food groups were mentioned as potential cause of an imbalanced terrain. Excessive use of protein, fat, or carbohydrates (starch) creates sludge in our blood stream that allows the proliferation of harmful microorganisms. This is a hint toward the fundamental Natural Law of Health known as "balance in all things." One key to health at the cellular level is a balance of protein, carbohydrates, fat, vitamins and minerals; along with the ions (electromagnetic force) for intracellular transport of nutrients and energy.

Simply put: what we eat and how we eat it is critically important to our health, longevity, and the quality of life we experience

NATURAL LAW: Everything exists in relation to its opposite. The conflict between opposites is the dynamic of life, and establishes an environment for balance.

both at this moment and in the future. We must learn how to remove dietary obstacles that block our bodies' ability to heal. We must learn how to have a nourishing diet that brings out our best, and fully supports our life endeavors. In this capacity, diet is a tool to loving more, experiencing more, being more of who we truly are. The next few chapters will present key insights to improving health through the missing elements of dietary factors. These elements are missing because, in many people's zeal to lose weight, they forget to simultaneously build their health.

When you get your FitTest results, you'll be shown how to design your ratios of macro-nutrients to activate your fat-burning mechanism to help you shed your unwanted weight. Part Two will make you a master of macro-nutrients so you can dine with ease and pleasure.

Part Two

Maximizing Macro-Nutrients: Your Key to Fat Burning Acceleration

CHAPTER SEVEN

The Seesaw Play Of The Macro-Nutrients

Seeds are quickened in the earth's dark night;
Plants spring green in vibrant air and light;
Fruits are ripened by the strong sun's might;
So quickens the soul in the heart's warm deep;
So flourishes the spirit in the wide world's keep;
So ripen human powers for God to reap.
- Table Grace, Rudolph Steiner

Here we begin our discussion on the macro-nutrients: protein, fats, and carbohydrate. Because, traditionally, this type of nutritional information is more academically oriented, many people find it ho-hum-boring. I understand. How can molecules compare with an exciting spy thriller or passionate romance novel? Because these particular macro-nutrient molecules are the alphabet of our diets and we want to spell two phrases — "fat-loss" and "optimal health" — I'll do my best to get tomes of text condensed down to the bare essentials.

Macronutrients are your alphabet that spells 'fat loss' when configured for that hormonal communication.

This introduction will provide a simple, graphic illustration of the relationships among the macro-nutrients so you'll know exactly what you are doing as you commit to re-sculpting your physique and improving your health with the FitTest and *The Weight Is Over* Program. The three macro-nutrient chapters are arranged so that you can use them as a quick-reference guide. All you need to do is learn a few facts and gain some insights from the ancient wisdom and you'll be able to prosper wherever you are.

What we eat becomes woven into the fabric of our bodies. Our diets become both the woof and warp of our tissue integrity. What are your threads? Recreational fluff or strong, bright fibers? A wonderful aspect of your body is its inherent ability to change or adapt. You can start now and reweave your health. It won't be long before every cell in your body rejoices in having its nutritional needs met. Happy cells mean long life.

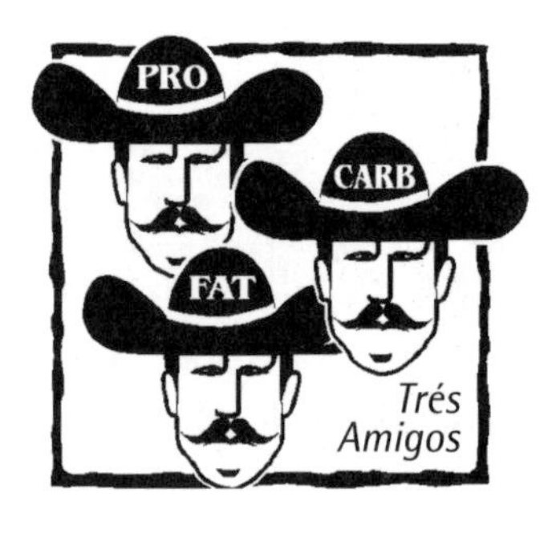

An interesting relationship exists between the macro-nutrients. Each holds an importance that the others can't do without for very long. Not only are these nutrients important for the fiber of our bodies, they are involved with other, complex hormonal activities. They function as a team to form the basis of our metabolic stability.

- Protein is the leader of the team. Too little and the body lacks direction and tissue strength. Too much and the body suffers from lack of helpful input.
- Fat is the hub. Both carbohydrates and protein need the fats to complete their hormonal missions.
- Carbohydrate is the fuel specialist. Too much and we experience the danger of a figurative explosion in weight. Too little and the body runs low on energy.

In a balanced system, these *trés amigos* set the foundation for our health. Whenever a person has the **wrong ratios of macronutrients,** side effects will occur.

- With *too much protein and not enough carbohydrate*, ketosis occurs. This is not necessarily a bad thing, since the body can burn ketone bodies as energy. In fact, the more the body burns ketones, the faster fat loss will occur, so a mild, controllable ketosis is a good fat-burning position. This can occur without the side effects and concerns of a high ketosis "crash" diet.

- A diet that is *too high in fat* can cause weight gain as the body stores the extra fat. It also causes metabolic sluggishness and mental fatigue.

- You already know the side effects of a diet that is *too high in carbohydrate* – insulin dominated metabolism and all its possible impediments to proper health.

The summary – again, a **balance of macro-nutrients** is the key to optimal hormonal response.

Picture a seesaw. On one end is carbohydrate: on the other end is protein. Fat is the hub. If the seesaw teeters toward carbohydrate, the insulin response can cause fat storage. If the seesaw totters toward protein, then the metabolism can burn fat via the glucagon hormonal response.

illus. 1

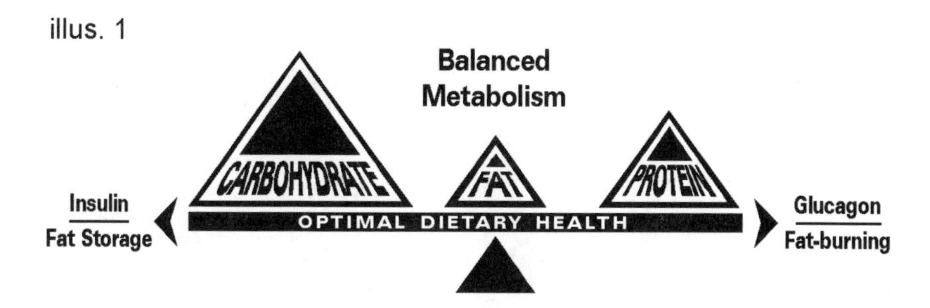

If the diet tips a little too much toward carbohydrate (illus. 2), fat storage can occur.

illus. 2

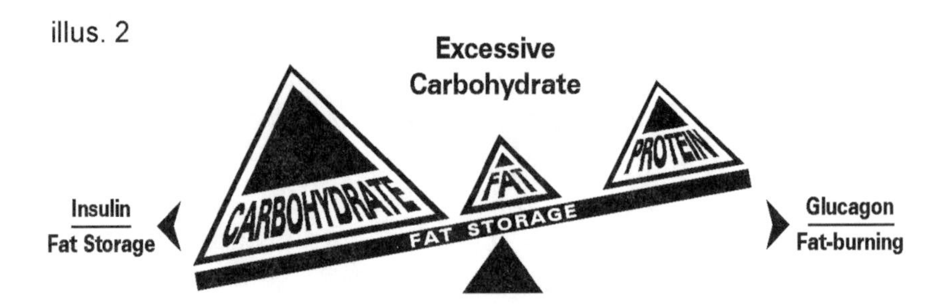

If it tips a little toward protein (illus. 3), then the fat burning mechanism is activated.

illus. 3

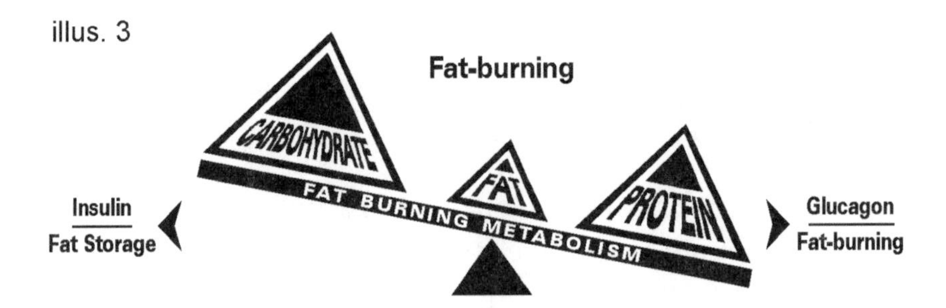

There is a further extreme to the seesaw. If it tips way too far toward carbohydrate (illus. 4), then glucose problems occur. If it tips way too far toward protein (illus. 5), then ketosis can occur, which rapidly burns fat for energy.

illus. 4

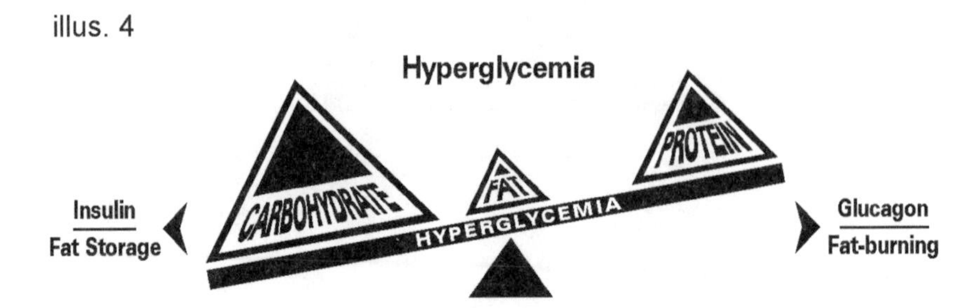

illus. 5

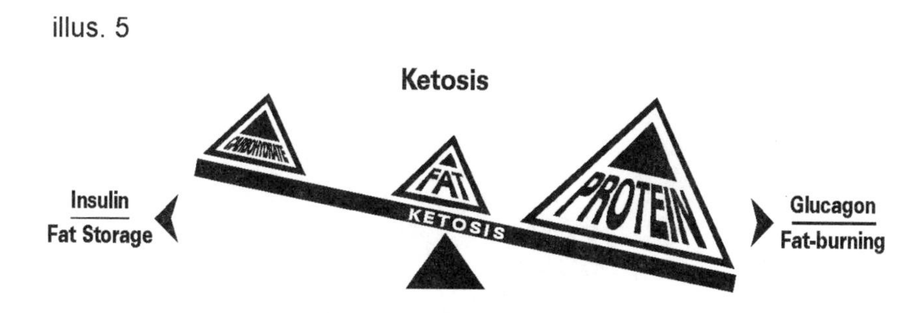

Just to include all options, if there is too much fat (illus. 6), then the seesaw ShiftsLeft to favor the storage of fat.

illus. 6

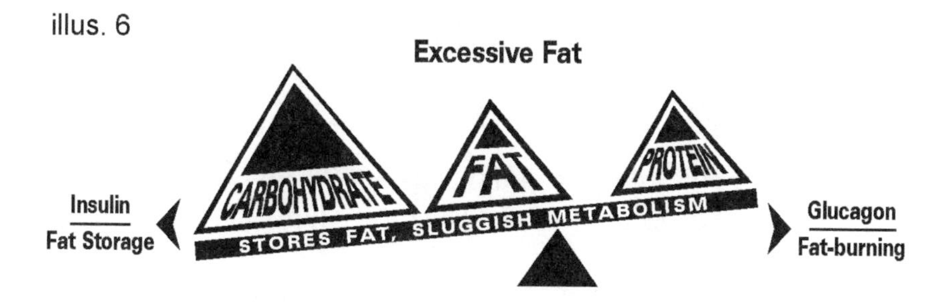

Let's make examples of some diets. Here is a graphic portrait of the high carbohydrate, low protein, low fat diet (illus. 7), sometimes called the "healthy heart diet". Look how it resembles Illustration 2, except there's even less fat, which makes this plan even more detrimental to nutritional health.

illus. 7

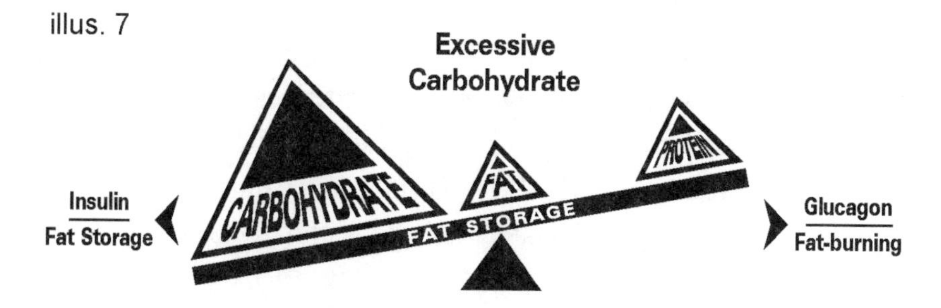

Finally, here is *The Weight Is Over* Program (illus. 8). It tips the seesaw gently to the fat burning side.

illus. 8

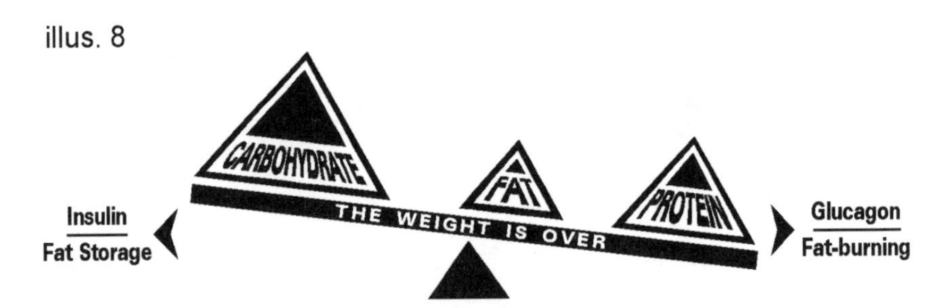

"The Weight is Over" Fat Burning Plan.
The degree the see-saw shifts right
is the degree of fat burning desired.

After *The Weight Is Over* Program helps you obtain the desired results, you will simply adjust your diet back to Illustration 1, *The Balanced Metabolism* to live long and prosper.

With these images to help us understand the role of the macro-nutrients, let's jump in and learn about these powerful tools that will bring us mastery over what we eat so we can live the life of our dreams.

The Macro-Nutrients

Armed with the grading scale of the 12 Optimal Nutrition Factors, let's learn about the three macro-nutrients. Let's first focus on one of the big wheels within wheels issues. We can balance our metabolisms (hormonal response to food) with a balance of macro-nutrients. We can also balance our metabolisms with the highest quality macro-nutrients, and gain the dynamic benefits of genuinely improved health. Once this "plate" is spinning properly, many metabolic processes necessary for optimal health fall into place. First, we'll take a quick look at a scientific basis for custom designing the big spinning plate of macro-nutrient balance in your weight picture. That knowledge will help you find a smoother pathway to the physique you desire. Let's become more familiar with the three macro-nutrients (protein, fats, and carbohydrates.) We will separate the beneficial from the detrimental, and learn how to adjust our diets to ShiftRight – where a more optimal degree of health awaits us.

For our purposes here, the intricacies of macro-nutrient metabolic pathways are unnecessary and laborious. We'll not discuss the roles of the various amino acids, how carbohydrates are processed into glucose, and the molecular structure of omega 3, 6, and 9 fatty acid molecules. This type of conversation is well covered in *Eating Energy*, where I have endeavored to communicate such topics in a way that everyone who is interested can understand and learn.

Here, we'll focus on the basic understanding of the macro-nutrients, so you'll know exactly what weight and health benefits await you when you look down at your plate and see the salad, the broccoli, the fish, the beans, the olive, the avocado, and so forth. On the other side of the coin, you'll see the high risk, skull-and-crossbones items that your health would appreciate that you avoid. Then, you will be able to make the right choice, or the right compromise, or at least a clear decision that you are taking a risk.

Every food has its pros and cons. A secret of good nutrition is a full and varied diet. Of course, you must have the pros outweigh the cons.

Statistics show that most people eat only around thirty foods. Take a moment and make a list of your primary foods – the ones you buy every week. You may be surprised on how few foods you are basing your nutrition. One goal of Part Two of this book is to introduce you to a greater variety of foods so you can expand your nutrition base. One of the basic premises of nutrition is that no one food is perfect in and of itself for all people in all phases of life. We need to provide our bodies a broad base of nutrients by eating a wide variety of foods. Every food, other than breast milk for an infant, has its pros and cons. This is so critically important a concept that I'll repeat it.

This means that even the super-great health foods have down sides. It also means that there can be some virtue in whole foods labeled "bad". With no one, natural food being all-perfect, or all bad, perhaps we can seek an understanding of dietary moderation and variety. Here are some examples of food pros and cons:

- Some people say, "Eat spinach to be strong like Popeye." Others say not to eat spinach because it can form kidney stones. Some say raw spinach has great virtues as a kidney cleanser. Others say cooked spinach has free oxalic acid that will bind calcium. When a whole, natural food becomes controversial, just use it moderately. A little spinach in a salad periodically will provide good nutrition, and any detrimental possibilities will all come out in the wash. That's Nature's way. Problems can potentially occur if a person lived on spinach juice for two weeks. That's an extreme use of a food. As with many foods, raw is better than cooked. With a moderate approach, we won't run screaming in fear when we find spinach in our omelet. Instead, we'll enjoy the benefits of a full and varied diet. Oftentimes, I tell the avid health-nuts to relax, enjoy, and don't worry about splitting hairs on smaller issues. More often than not, they don't really matter in the big picture.

- How about all the controversy regarding the egg? Some say it's one of Nature's greatest protein foods. Others say it is bad because it contains cholesterol. Assuming we are talking about a farm-fresh, free-range, naturally-fed chicken egg, the benefits far outweigh any concerns when the facts are put on the scale. But this is in context of eggs as a part of a full and varied diet, not someone eating 20 hard-boiled eggs a day and nothing else.

- Sometimes super foods (foods renowned for reputed health benefits) turn out to be not such a good idea when taken to extreme. My files contain stories of a person who lived on carrot juice and became diabetic, of a lady who ate large quantities of blue green algae and was found to have it live and viable in her intestines, of a fruitarian (only eats fruit) who developed muscle atrophy and lost her hair.

- Some people "throw the baby out with the bathwater." A man who avoided all fat via a self-styled "Pritikin Diet" developed nerve afflictions and eczema, only to have it go away **in days** when he added flaxseed oil and grapeseed oil to his diet. A vegetarian avoided all meat, went on a high-carbohydrate, high processed-sugar diet, and developed the beginning rash of beriberi – a thiamine (B-vitamin deficiency.)

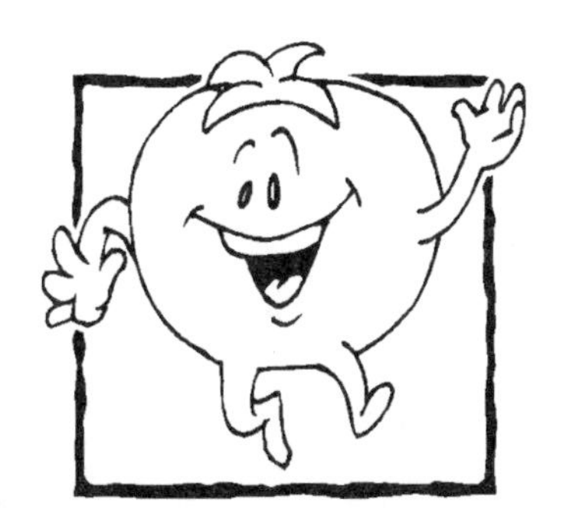

Here we find the case for dietary variety and freedom. Variety is the spice of life. Freedom allows more choices. Endeavor to expand your basic thirty foods to fifty or more. Expand your diet for variety of tastes and nutrients.

- Instead of eating broccoli three times a week, add some cauliflower and green beans to the medley.
- Try some jicama slices with lime juice for a snack.
- If you shy away from squash, put a raw slice in your salad.

- If you eat chicken five times a week, substitute in some fish or a game bird.
- If you eat a lot of russet potatoes, try a yam.
- Add herbs to your foods. Fresh basil, chopped rosemary, or a pinch of sage adds not only exotic flavors, but also other oils and nutrients to the standard fare. Note: buy your herbs and spices at the health food store to avoid the nuclear-irradiated "dead" herbs often sold at the grocery stores even though "irradiation" is often not mentioned on the label.

Use the following macro-nutrient chapters to identify new foods that you don't normally eat, and introduce them into your diet. Begin a phase of culinary adventure and bring new foods to your plate. You'll improve your nutrition and probably find some wonderful new friends. *Bon appetite!*

CHAPTER EIGHT

Protein's Role in Fat Burning and Health

With respect to food and nutrition...the whole is greater than the sum of the parts
- Dr. Royal Lee

Let's examine the critical role of protein in health and weight loss. Protein is the key to your weight optimization plan, the macro-nutrient that leads the way. Carbohydrates are "cheap and easy" to bring into the diet. Fats often accompany proteins and the primary preoccupation regarding fats is to avoid the ugly fats and include the beneficial fats daily because they prime your fat-burning pathways. Nutrition is a team effort, but protein plays the pivotal role and is the leader of the team. With proper management of protein, the key nutritional issues automatically fall into place.

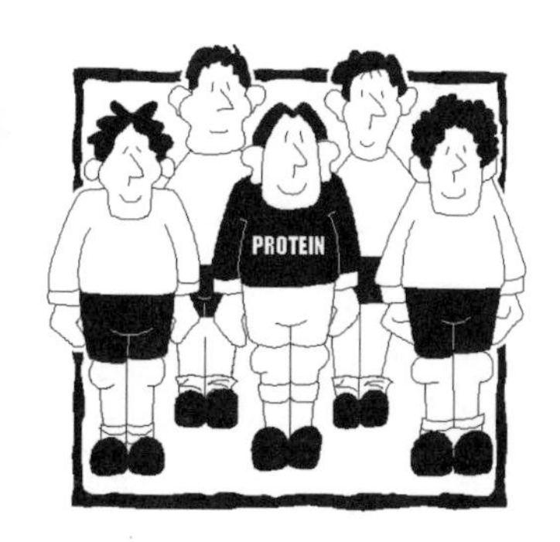

What Is Protein?

The word, "*protein,*" means "of primary importance" and protein is an *essential* food meaning we must have an external, dietary source for it. We can't live without it. Protein's basic structural unit, the *amino acid*, is the building block of life because it is essential for growth and repair of every part of the body. The most important proteins are the nucleo-proteins, amino acids that are small enough for the cells to use for repair and energy.

What Is The Role Of Protein In The Body?

To emphasize the point that protein is of primary importance, consider this. Proteins are responsible for:

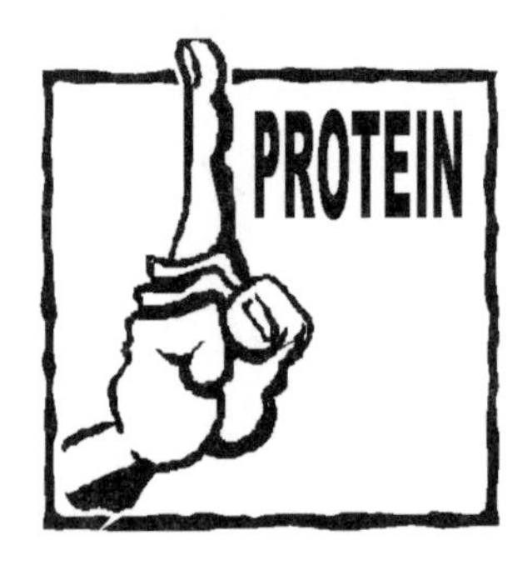

- Hemoglobin (carries oxygen in the blood)
- Hormones (metabolism, tissue repair, blood sugar balance, etc.)
- Immunoglobins (protection from bacteria, fungus, virus)
- Enzymes (digestion, assimilation, and utilization of food, anti-aging)
- Neurotransmitters (feelings: joy, confidence, pain relief, sleep, sex drive)
- Muscle contractions (ability to walk, run, breathe, have a heart beat)
- RNA and DNA (the genetic codes that run everything)
- Bone and teeth formation
- Intestinal tissue integrity (ability to absorb nutrients and eliminate undesirable substances)
- Maintaining body fluid balance
- Transportation of vitamins and minerals
- Transportation of beneficial ions (bio-energy) to the cells for ATP (energy) synthesis

How Do Proteins Help You ShiftRight Into Fat-Burning?

Here's how to shift your diet to the right regarding protein nutrition and use it to activate your fat-burning mechanism. The first few items are self-explanatory. The last few items are summarized here, then more material is presented on that topic later in this chapter. Once you get the hang of it, protein nutrition will be a piece of cake! [Just kidding.]

Dietary proteins form the hub of fat-burning nutrition.

ShiftRight Health and Fat Loss Tips

Eat Breakfast Like a King: Have a *The Weight Is Over* balanced protein meal early in the day to help stabilize blood sugar and to allow effective digestion, assimilation, absorption, and utilization during waking hours when the body is in motion and the lymphatic transport system is flowing. No more toast and coffee or donuts for breakfast! Have a truly nutritious breakfast.

Supper Like A Pauper: Eat lightly in the evening because it takes several hours for protein digestion to occur and a big digestive work-load interferes with sleep. Small amounts of food will tide you over until breakfast and keep you in the fat-burning mode. The smaller suppers allow your body time to detoxify and repair itself during the sleep cycle – the time it does this the best – because it is not preoccupied with digesting a heavy meal all night. [Note for *Pro-Vita! Plan* fans: The rule about minimizing protein foods late in the day is suspended during this *therapeutic* dietary approach to fat loss.]

Digestion: Avoid eating concentrated proteins with high glycemic sugars and starches such as bacon and jelly, eggs and a bagel. That combination results in poor digestion and elevated insulin response. Instead, support your digestion with a small salad or lightly steamed vegetables.

If your digestion is weak, it is best to take a digestive supplement. "All diseases start in the stomach" is an old naturopathic aphorism that refers to the importance of digestion. This is discussed further in *Your Liver ... Your Lifeline* (Tips, 1990)

Exercise to circulate proteins throughout the body and to build more lean tissue mass. Lean muscle burns fat. As you build muscle, you'll accelerate fat-loss. Further, exercise circulates the lymphatic fluid which is your garbage disposal system and will help you remove partially-processed fat molecules called "ketones". The more your remove, the faster your body burns fat. Right now, schedule some time each day for exercise – a walk, a bike ride, a work out, a sport.

Include Essential Fatty Acids (EFA's): Include a small amount of high-quality oil to prime the hormonal responses into the fat-burning metabolism. I'll explain this later, in the "Fats" chapter. Beneficial EFA's can be included in your diet with olives, olive oil or grape seed oil on a small salad, seeds, and nuts; and with dietary supplements.

Minimize High-Stress snacks: Refrain from eating large amounts of complex proteins (raw nuts, textured vegetable protein, peanuts) by themselves as snacks because, being difficult to digest, they deplete the digestive processes. Instead, combine low-stress proteins with raw vegetables for snacks (such as celery stuffed with tahini or a little cashew butter, balanced food bars, balanced protein powders, cottage cheese dips) while you are activating your fat-burning mechanism. Combining low stress proteins with vegetables for snacks will maximize your *The Weight Is Over* program and will keep you in the fat-burning dimension.

Assimilation, Micro-Nutrients, and pH: One practice helps with **all three** of these topics, and more. *Always use raw or lightly steamed vegetables with proteins.* The nutrient-factors in vegetables help with the assimilation of amino acids, provide much needed vitamins, minerals, and trace minerals, as well as fiber. They provide the basis for the alkaline mineral reserve your body needs as a foundation of nutritional health. Further, they buffer the acids of protein, making them safe and gentle on the acid/alkaline (pH) swings of the body. Eating raw or lightly steamed vegetables with every meal provides your body with what it needs to metabolize protein. Vegetables provide the necessary enzymes, fiber, nutrients, water, and bio-energy that help proteins impart more of their healing potential.

Longevity Advice: *Part One.* Have raw and lightly steamed vegetables with every meal. *Part Two.* Yes, that means with breakfast.

Balance of Macro-Nutrients: Use the right amount of protein – not too much, not too little. This information is provided with your FitTest results. You must have the right amount of protein in comparison to carbohydrates and fat in your diet to harness the hormone glucagon to burn fat. This provides the fat-burning *ratio* you need for a balanced, fat-burning metabolism. Further, the right quantity prevents the loss of muscle mass needed to burn more fat. More details about this topic are covered later in this chapter in "How Much Protein Do You Need Every Day?"

PROTEIN ECONOMY: Regarding protein nutrition, there is strength in variety.

Provide complete proteins over the course of the day to avoid the body having to make up complete proteins from the muscles or lymph-pool. This happens automatically with *The Weight Is Over* Plan, and we'll discuss this further in the "What Are The Protein Foods?" section later in this chapter.

Bio-Availability: Don't over cook. Heat alters the viability of amino acids. For example, charred meat and hard-boiling of eggs makes high-stress proteins compared to low-stress proteins produced by lighter cooking of protein foods. Textured vegetable proteins have been heat-altered in the processing and become high-stress foods. Use enough heat to cook the food, but endeavor to cook only to the degree the food actually needs. Much detail about how to cook foods to help keep them low-stress is found in *Eating Energy*.

It's not the protein content of a food that matters, but the *bio-availability* of the protein, i.e., what we can digest, assimilate, complete, humanize, and convert to complete amino acids and nucleo-proteins and eliminate by-products of that sets the standard of our health. Any food that can't go through these processes smoothly is a **high-stress food**. Keep reading. This subject will be explained further in sections of text about Biological Value and Low Stress Proteins.

Proteins are the key to rejuvenation. Only the high quality proteins can build a high quality state of cellular health.

Quality: Use high-quality, low-stress proteins listed later in this chapter. Most weight loss diets don't emphasize the **quality** of the protein used. Any protein will serve to initiate the fat-burning hormones for fat-loss, but only the low-stress (high quality) proteins will build high quality tissue.

How Much Protein Do You Need Every Day?

There is a very wide range of grams of protein needed by individuals for optimal health. This range is highly debated and there are a wide variety of opinions.

- Some researchers say this range is from 25% to 50% of total caloric intake.
- Others say it's a percentage between .6 and .9 grams of protein/kilogram of body weight.

- Still others say it's a percentage of lean body mass.

After choosing a method of calculating, we have to accommodate our activity level and a host of other factors. What does this really mean? The range of protein needed to sustain life and adequate health is very wide. This is why there are so many high- as well as low- protein regimens that all claim success. The range of protein for optimal health, though smaller than the survival range, is still wide enough for a variety of dietary lifestyles.

Protein is critical for optimal fat-burning:
1. The right ratio of protein compared to carbohydrate and fat.
2. The right amount of protein to prevent muscle loss when the body starts burning fat.

During a weight loss regimen, maintaining optimal dietary protein intake is much more important than during times of "just living" because the fat-burning metabolic pathways are dependent on the proper ratio of protein to other foods. It is important to protect the muscles from losing weight. This is why, for weight loss, measurements of lean body mass are taken and the rules include eating a more exact amount of protein daily.

For an optimal fat-loss program, without muscle-loss, you must be in the ballpark of optimal protein intake, and the job *of The Weight Is Over* Program is to get you a terrific seat in the ballpark. Here is where science can help you get in the ballpark much more easily than trial and error or attempting a "one-size-fits-all" formula. Calculating lean body mass and applying it to dietary intake of protein can help you get in the ballpark by helping you ensure you are getting enough protein to make the whole program work. How to calculate lean body mass is courteously provided with the FitTest so you can plan your fat-burning program more accurately.

Individually-defined factors governing protein requirements:

Body weight
Lean muscle mass
Activity level (sedentary vs. athletic)
Strength of the stomach's hydrochloric acid (digestion)
Strength of the pancreas's proteolytic enzymes (digestion)
Emotional state (supportive or inhibitive of digestion)
Effectiveness of mastication (chewing)
Combination of foods eaten (enhance or inhibit digestion)
Time of day eaten (enzyme availability)
Preparation (raw, cooked)
Pregnancy (requirements increase)

What Are The Protein Foods?

Protein foods are as varied in structure as the many vast differences in life forms on Earth. Some ratios of amino acids comprising a protein molecule match the body's optimal requirements and are called *complete proteins*. Other proteins (called *incomplete proteins*,) while high in amino acid chains, lack essential amino acids. The body will have to add amino acids to these structures before it can use them effectively. Generally, complete proteins are ones that have been synthesized by an animal such as meat, egg, and milk, and incomplete proteins are the vegetable proteins. The body can take incomplete proteins and put them together to make complete proteins provided it has the essential amino acids to do this. It can get those essential amino acids from other foods eaten (if they are inherent in those foods), or can sacrifice its own lymphatic pool or even muscle tissue to make them complete and able to perform for the body's needs.

The following three tables categorize protein foods according to the macro-nutrient in which they are found. (Not all foods listed here are optimal, low stress foods.)

Primarily Protein.

Protein is the highest of the three macro-nutrients.

Beef (Veal)	Pork
Cheese	Protein Powder
Chicken	Shellfish (Crab, Lobster, Mussels, Oysters, Scallops, Shrimp)
Eggs	Tempeh
Fish / Seafood	Tofu
Fowl (Duck, Cornish Game Hens, Goose, Dove, Pheasant)	Turkey
Goat	Whey Protein
Lamb (Sheep)	

Fat-Protein.

Foods that have the largest ratio of macro-nutrient as fat, include significant protein content and are often used as sources of dietary protein.

Cream Cheese

Nuts (Almond, Brazil, Cashew, Chestnut, Filbert, Hazelnut, Macadamia, Pecan, Peanut, Pine Nut, Pistachio, Walnut)

Seeds (Pumpkin, Sesame, Squash, Sunflower)

Carbohydrate-Protein.

Foods that are predominately carbohydrates, but contain a significant amount of protein, often used as a source of protein.

Asparagus	Lentils
Beans	Milk
Beet Leaf	Quinoa
Bulgar wheat	Soy
Broccoli	Sprouts (Sunflower, Mung, Alfalfa, Chia, Soy, etc.)
Brussels Sprouts	Yogurt
Chlorella	

We must ensure that our bodies receive a complete array of amino acids and are not lacking in any of the *essential* amino acids. The liver can assemble many of the amino acids that the body needs, but there are 10 (some researchers say 9) essential amino acids that must come from food. When these are provided in our diet, they prevent the breakdown of our muscles to complete what our food is lacking. We need our muscles to burn fat, not make up complete protein structures. Further, we need protein to build our muscles (carbohydrates and fat will not build muscle). Therefore, complete proteins are a secret to optimal weight loss as well as optimal lean body mass.

Complete proteins are a law of economy. Cells require complete proteins and we live and die at the cellular level. This means more energy and a longer life.

Complete protein structures are found in a variety of unlikely places. Fruit often contains complete proteins – just a tiny amount. Many vegetables contain complete proteins – again just a small amount. Many "protein" foods are not complete, such as most seeds and nuts; yet sesame seeds are complete, but limited. The general rule regarding protein nutrition is to eat a variety of foods so that deficiencies and imbalances are less likely to occur. Again, variety embraces the profound nutritional principle – *it all comes out in the wash.*

Another way to derive complete proteins is by combining incomplete but complimentary protein foods over the course of the day. This method involves some work from the body, but it presents the feasibility of vegetable protein diets – first, because the combination can increase the *biological value*, and second, because, with some work, the body can construct complete proteins when the various components are provided over the course of a day or two.

The Biological Value Of Proteins

You might be interested to know that Nutritional Science has provided a method to determine the biological value (BV) of proteins. It's called "Net Protein Utilization". These tables are based on the egg because Science determined that an egg was a perfect protein and assigned the perfect score of 100. Later, whey protein was "discovered" and found to have a higher biological value than egg, so the scale now exceeds 100. (If I had been asked, I would have established human breast milk, which is 80% whey, as the benchmark for human beings.) The target range for effective proteins is 70 and above. The following table examines the completeness of protein foods in an attempt to show how much of a protein food can be made available for use in the body.

Protein Biological Values (BV) or Net Protein Utilization (NPU)

Whey, cow milk, goat milk	104
Egg	100
Cow's milk	92
Meat (wild game)	82
Beef	80
Chicken, fowl	80
Fish	79
Casein	77
Soy ferments	74
Potato	71
Rice	59
Wheat	54
Beans	49
Target for Effective Protein	**70 and above**

All proteins are not created equal. Proteins are not the same, despite the scientific view that ignores the viability of proteins to transport and impart electromagnetic energy. *Quality* is important and carries an intrinsic value. A protein's *true biological value* depends on

- how available its nutrients are for the body, and
- how much biochemical and electromagnetic energy it can provide to the body.

Therefore, the scientific biological value of a protein food is not the only test the food must pass to earn a positive rating on the *Eating Energy 12 Optimal Food Factors*, but it does show us the potential protein foods that can play a role in protein nutrition. The following table lists some of the factors that determine a protein's bio-availability.

Food-defined factors governing protein utilization

Quality of protein
Quantity of protein
Agricultural methods to produce food (chemical vs. organic)
Bio-energy of food (freshness, processing, heat alteration, structure of amino acids, etc.)
Anti-proteolytic factors inherent (food-enzymes that inhibit protein digestion)
Fat content of food (fat defined by nature, or by force feeding)
Carbohydrate content of food (determines digestion effectiveness)
Completeness of the essential amino acids
Presence of protein-enhancing vegetables

Low-Stress Protein Foods

For The Weight Is Over edge, here is a table of low-stress proteins. These foods have a high biological availability. This list of protein foods has served thousands of people well during their fat-loss and dietary regimens. Both vegetarian and non-vegetarian proteins are listed here. The common element is that high stress protein foods have been omitted and are shown at the end of the list in an explanatory paragraph. Omitted (high-stress) proteins should not form the basis of a person's diet. They can be used occasionally if necessary.

Protein Foods

(Biologically Available)

Low Stress Proteins

Abalone

Beans (organic, fresh, sprouted, cooked without boiling as in a crock pot) aduki, black, kidney, lima, lentils, mung, navy, pinto, white, yellow

Beet Greens (organic, fresh)

Black-eyed peas (organic, soaked, cooked below boil)

Cheese (organic, goat, sheep and cow cheese, not heated [cooked])

Chicken, (organic, free-range, without skin)

Chlorella (sea algae, grown mercury-free)

Clam

Coconut milk, green, young (the clear milk gel, not the mature coconut, which is mostly fat)

Conch (sea mussel, mollusk)

Cornish game hen (organic)

Cottage cheese (organic raw milk from sheep, goat, cow)

Crab (especially king crab)

Crawfish

Dove (game bird)

Duck (game bird)

Eggs (chicken, organic, free-range or yard, cooked low heat)

Escargot (snail)

Feta cheese (organic sheep, goat)

Fish (ocean, cold, deep water, fresh)

Arctic char, flounder, grouper, haddock, halibut, mahi-mahi, monkfish, orange roughy, salmon, snapper, sea bass, sole, tuna (fresh), wahoo, whiting, yellowtail

Frog legs

Gelatin (Grayslake, 180 bloom, can be used in soup)

Goose (organic, free range)

Lobster

Miso (fermented grain-paste for soup)
Mussel, green lipped
Nutmilks (organic, soaked overnight, blended in water) almond, cashew
Octopus
Peas (organic)
Pheasant (game bird)
Pine Nuts (mostly beneficial fat)
Quail (game bird)
Scallops
Seeds, germinated (soaked) pumpkin, sunflower, squash, chia, sesame
Seed Milks (pumpkin, sunflower, squash, sesame)
Sesame Tahini (Sesame seed butter)
Shrimp
Soy ferments (miso, tempeh, natto, soy sauce)
Sprouts (alfalfa, chia, flax, mung, sunflower, flax)
Squib (game pigeon)
Squid
Tempeh (soy ferment)
Tofu
Turkey
Turtle (a red meat, but not high stress)
Whey (milk product)
Wild-rice (soaked, cooked below boil)
Yogurt (organic, raw goat and cow milk)

High Stress Proteins

For people who want to eat red meat (a medium to high-stress protein source largely due to the enhanced fat content of agricultural methods), commercial meats should be avoided. The best choices for red meat are water buffalo, bison, free-range ostrich, free-range emu, organically-grown sheep, goat, and wild game (elk, caribou, and various deer venisons). Pork is generally considered a high-stress meat due to the amount and structure of the fat accompanying it and its tendency for parasites; however, there are new debates in the nutrition community regarding this.

Some Major Protein Issues For Vegetarian Diets

An important conclusion can be drawn from the biological availability table. Larger volumes of protein foods are required in a plant-protein (vegetarian) diet than in a diet that includes animal protein foods. This means that a vegetarian will need to eat larger quantities of protein-rich vegetable foods such as seeds, nuts, miso, tofu, or will need to add whey, cheese, or eggs to attain the hormonal response of the fat-burning ratio.

Some vegetarian proteins are of high quality, some are of low quality. Some animal source proteins are of high quality, some are of low quality.

The discussion of vegetarian vs. non-vegetarian lifestyles is not germane to our topic of fat-burning. There are pros and cons to both points that fill many pages. Both vegetarians and non-vegetarians have problems with excessive fat gain. Both can activate their hormones to burn fat, though it is more difficult for the vegetarian because of the tendency to "carbotarian" meals. This book will discuss proteins from all sources that can initiate and sustain the fat-burning mechanism and provide ways for everyone to enjoy fat-weight loss. A discussion of the on-going controversy and the *Eating Energy* solution is reserved for the more lengthy format of the *Eating Energy* book.

How will vegetarians, people who eat no meat, succeed in losing weight when the vegetarian diet uses predominately carbohydrate foods and avoids the high and complete protein foods? Dr. Wheelwright used to say that he never met a true vegetarian. All he met were "carbotarians – people who lived on starch, not vegetables." He maintained that a true vegetarian would be a person who ate mostly vegetables as in broccoli, asparagus, cabbage, and so forth. Vegetarian fat-loss is more difficult and takes some planning, but it can be done. Some helpful hints for how a vegetarian can tip the scale toward protein balance is found in the next chapter, "Protein Health and Fat Loss Tips."

Conclusion

As an individual dedicated to optimal dietary health, I have experimented with every position on protein – high vs. low, meat vs. vegetable, complete vs. incomplete, as well as the middle-ground combinations. In so doing, I have tested the validity of the facts and myths, and separated the philosophies from the realities. Through it all, the overview of Natural Law and the *Eating Energy 12 Optimal Nutritional Factors* helped me synthesize some key insights, which I hope are helpful to you. Here they are in a nutshell:

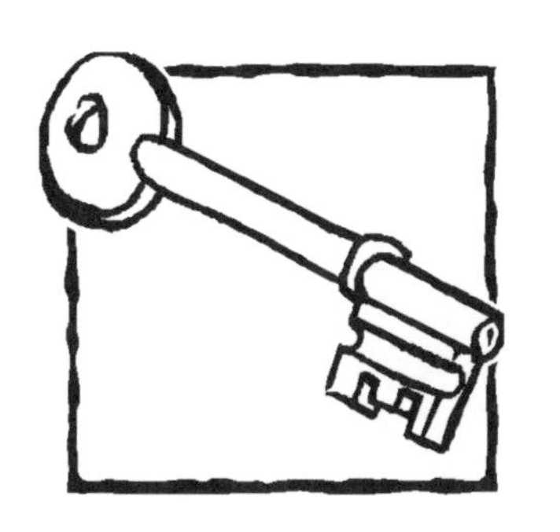

The issue of protein in the diet comes down to the simple factors of quality and quantity. **If we can eat the right amount of high quality proteins, in proper balance with other macro-nutrients, our health and our weight will greatly improve.**

This chapter has taught the essence of the many variables of protein nutrition. Ultimately, energy is the issue of fat-loss. The burning of fat alters the physique and provides a better metabolic energy for your life endeavors. Enjoy the process of re-designing your physique. It'll boost your self-confidence and build a more positive future.

CHAPTER NINE

Protein: Health and Fat Loss Tips

There is only cause of disease – congestion.
There is only one cure – circulation.
- Old Chinese Aphorism

I hope you can now take the information about protein and organize the hub of your fat-burning meals. After all that information, it really boils down to a few simple steps that pay enormous dividends to your health.

Health and Fat Loss Tips

1. For fat-loss, use the correct amount of protein and vegetable combinations for your meals.

2. Use a properly-balanced supplement (powder, bars) when you're in a hurry or you have a craving. Your individualized "proper balance" is what your FitTest results will help determine. You can check a supplement's label to see how its macro-nutrient ratios compare with your personal requirements.

Proteins and Bio-Energy

Here is a brief comment about the importance of proteins. Proteins are important carriers of the body's bio-energetic, or bio-magnetic energy. *Quality* proteins can carry and give up ions of energy (ch'i) for the free-circulation of energy. Nucleo proteins are the basis for RNA, from which a cell's mitochondria derives *adenosine triphosphate* (ATP). This is the spark of life in the cell, the fuel for cellular life and the battery for the bio-energetic field. ATP, a protein, powers the cell. **This is particularly important for athletes because ATP powers the muscles.** Poor-quality proteins absorb bio-energy and hold onto it, depleting free ions and preventing their free circulation. This causes congestion.

The Future Ain't What It Used To Be

Is it really a surprise that things change? As we age, our metabolisms change. We must adapt our diets to our current phase of life. This means we can't eat like a teenager when we're 50 years old. The human body goes through metabolic changes or cycles of life. We have to be willing to adapt, accept, and change with our bodies. This is Natural Law.

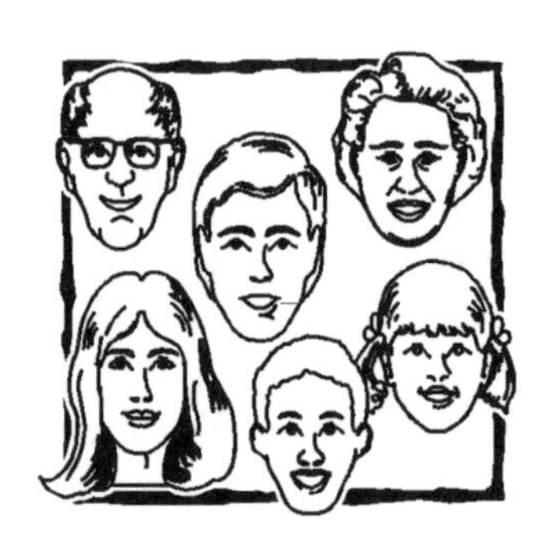

There are cycles of life. First is infancy-childhood – a phase marked by rapid growth. Pre-puberty is another time of mental, emotional, and physical changes. Next are the changes to adulthood. Later comes female and male menopause, and finally, the elder years. During these epochs of life, the body operates under different metabolisms, different hormonal cycles, and different acid/alkaline ranges. Each cycle is necessary and right. Each cycle is an inevitable part of life and is characterized by its unique power.

The diet that works best during the different cycles of life is one that fits the time. Children can process more carbohydrate than adults. As adults get older, they need to realize that their proper level of carbohydrate foods will change. Elderly people need more alkalizing foods (vegetables) than youngsters to offset the acid swing that contributes to osteoporosis, arthritis, and so forth.

When we eat the way we used to and don't change with the times, we will suffer the consequences of an improper diet. Hank Williams, Jr. sings about the changes of life and comments that his friends aren't rowdy any more, "Hangovers hurt more than they used to ..." For many people, this "eating in the past" produces weight gain. The equation regarding weight is simple. If you eat more than you need of any macro-nutrient, especially if you eat too many refined carbohydrates, you gain fat. What determines "too much" and the proper ratio is predominately age (cycle of life) and metabolism (assessed by FitTest). Middle-aged men often tell me in consultations, "I move a little slower. I can't do what I used to." They acknowledge that their bodies don't move like they did when their were teenagers. They don't run as fast, lift as much, or go as long. Yet, their diets often contain more food and "life's little pleasures" of candy, chips, beer, donuts, desserts. By now, I hope you can see how that simple mistake ends up as a "Homer Simpson" physique. It can also lead to chronic, degenerative disease.

If you see elements of yourself in this story, then your first step is to reduce the size of your meals and balance the macro-nutrients. Over a little time, your extended stomach will shrink and you will be perfectly satisfied with the smaller meals that are right for you. Buy a smaller plate and when its food is eaten, you're finished. Enjoy what you have and don't go back for seconds. This simple, virtually painless approach will help the future become what you dream, not what you dread.

Ketosis And The Diminished Appetite

For some people, a **low appetite** can occur when they switch to a high-protein weight-loss diet. As their body burns fat, a mild ketosis is induced. This is the state where the body feeds on itself to render fat (and proteins if they are lacking in the diet) into glucose. The by-products of this process can satisfy and lower the appetite because fat is being processed. If this occurs, nutritionists counsel people to continue eating, even though they are not hungry, because they must continue priming the fat-burning pump as well as protect their muscle mass.

As good as it sounds to have a low appetite and not be fighting hunger to lose weight, **the low appetite person must remember to eat to lose weight.**

The Weight Is Over Program does not induce a severe ketosis like medically-supervised liquid protein diets. It's neither necessary nor desirable. Instead, we first balance the diet, then shift it safely and gently into the fat-burning mode. You can *accelerate* your individualized plan simply by avoiding more of the refined carbohydrates. Conversely, you *will slow it down* when you tip your balance into too much carbohydrate.

Your fat-burning mechanism is only as active as your last meal dictates.

The reason high ketosis diets are medically supervised is that they have three drawbacks:

1. With the absence of carbohydrate in the diet, the body can choose to secrete insulin, due to the presence of *protein*, as a self-preservation directive. When this happens, fat loss is inhibited and people can have the same side effects as a high carbohydrate diet – low human growth hormone, muscle loss, and blood sugar fluctuations.
2. Excessive ketones in the body causes an activation of the enzyme inside the fat cells that make them hungry to store fat. The fat cells want to replace the fat they've lost.
3. Breaking the diet can cause rapid weight **regain** unless there is a careful plan.

After beginning *The Weight Is Over* Program, you can, with the help of the journal in Part 3, track your improvement. If you wish to accelerate your program, be sure you do not have any hidden sugars in your diet. Read labels and weed them out. This will accelerate your fat loss. The more you remove refined and processed carbohydrates from your diet, the faster you will lose fat. By eating raw and lightly steamed vegetables with every meal, you will keep a safe level of carbohydrates in your diet so your body burns fat without sacrificing muscle mass or entering a state of excessive ketosis.

Helpful Hints For Vegetarian Dieters

Here's how a vegetarian can tip the scale toward protein balance:

First, Vegetarians should cut off the excessively rich carbohydrates.

- Stop eating refined sugar, sweets, and high-sweet foods (desserts, honey, sodas, dates, raisins, candy).
- Stop eating high glycemic starches (processed cereals, micro-wave cooked or baked potatoes, instant oatmeal, instant rice or potato dishes, beer, pasta, puffed rice, corn, wheat products, bananas, carrot juice, breads).

Next, Vegetarians should use low glycemic foods instead of the excessively rich carbohydrates.

- Eat vegetables and fruit.
- Some people (approx. 25%) can handle small amounts of *al dente* low-glycemic grains (barley pearls, quinoa, whole rye, whole oats, spelt, amaranth, etc.). Less cooking means less glucose-induction.

Then, Vegetarians should add a combination of vegetarian protein foods:

- Add seeds and nuts (preferably soaked in water overnight), miso, tofu, tempeh. [If an ovo/lacto diet is acceptable, use eggs, cottage cheese, feta cheese.]
- Supplement protein intake with protein food bars and/or protein powders mixed in water. Strict vegetarians will have to use soy or rice proteins. Lacto-vegetarians should use whey protein powder, or soy/whey combinations during their fat-reduction program.

Next comes the exciting area of Fats. Yes, you will learn that you can, and, in fact, *should*, be eating fats to lose weight.

CHAPTER TEN

Fats' Fabulous Role in Fat-Burning

It is better to be beautiful than to be good.
But it is better to be good than ugly.
- Oscar Wilde

The Awesome Power Of Fat

The study of fats (lipids) is one of the most exciting areas of nutritional research today because of the healing, therapeutic and disease-preventative properties of fat. As nutritional and medical researchers delve deeper into the mysteries of nutrition and health, the importance of fats skyrockets.

In proportion to the incredible healing and health-sustaining properties of fats is controversy. More than any other nutrient, fats have been involved with misrepresentation of research, cover-ups, and overt manipulation of public information by those with profits to gain. The stakes are high, and knowledge is power. Join me, now, and learn to master fats in your diet.

Fats are a two-edged sword. With one swoop they heal and sustain. With the reverse arc, they kill.

Contrary to the undeserved bad name extolled in the media, fats are vitally important to our health. They are one of the three macro-nutrients upon which our entire health picture revolves. Fats are the hub around which proteins and carbohydrates balance. Without the "beautiful" and "good" fats, a person cannot be healthy. But, with the "ugly" fats, health is destroyed and life spans are shortened.

You must eat fat to activate the body's fat-burning mechanism.

At the beginning of this topic, let me emphasize again the beneficial, vital importance of fats because too many people equate fat with something that harms our health and makes us fat. Did you know the following fat facts?

- **You have to eat fat (the essential fatty acids) in order to lose excess fat.** Essential fatty acids increase your metabolic rate, which, in this case, means that the "beautiful" fats speed up your ability to burn fat and metabolize glucose. This means you burn more fat and store less.

- **There are fats that protect your cardiovascular system.** They actually protect your arteries, maintain proper blood pressure, and lower cholesterol.

- **Fats control your ability to fight cancer and prevent allergies.** Fats have a strong influence over the immune system and its ability to do its job properly. Underactive or ignorant immune systems can let cancer cells develop. Overactive or hyper immune systems can fight unnecessarily and cause allergy reactions and auto-immune diseases. The tendency to immune system imbalances is, in part, regulated by fats.

- **Fat also controls the combustion of carbohydrate. Fat is the key to improving athletic performance.** Massimo Testa, trainer of American cyclist Lance Armstrong states: *"You need good fat-burning for the aerobic engine. But the key to building a fat-burning system is to include the right fats in the diet."*

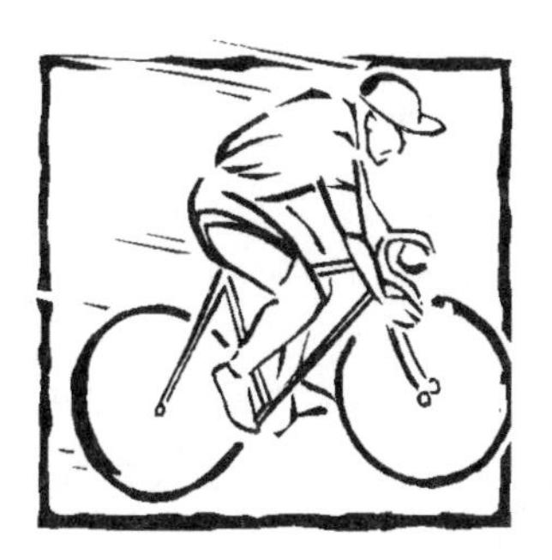

You Mean Fats Aren't Bad For Me?

Natural fats are not "bad." They are a necessary nutrient and health is dependent on them. Three factors determine if a particular fat is helpful or harmful to health.

To be healthful, a fat should be:

1. balanced within its own family of lipids (fats),
2. a high-quality, beautiful or good fat,
3. in balance with the other two macro-nutrients, carbohydrate and protein.

Conversely, there are three reasons that fats become killers:

1. *They are out of balance within their own family.* The imbalance in our current diet is too much omega-6 (vegetable oils) and not enough omega-3 oils (flaxseed oil, fish oils.)

2. *Fats are of low quality.* Low quality "ugly" fats are created when they are processed, (exposed to heat, light, oxygen,) hydrogenated and preserved. These fats cause major damage to the cardiovascular and immune systems. Also, some commercial oils contain enzyme inhibitors and toxic residues (such as nickel or pesticides) that make them less than optimal.

3. *The amount of fats is not balanced with the other macro-nutrients.* Fats become a health issue when there is too little or too much fat compared to protein and carbohydrate. *An imbalance or deficiency* can shut down the body's produc-

tion of the *eicosanoids* (the super micro-hormones regulating our life processes at the cellular level) that manage major body activities such as the storage of fat. *Too much dietary fat* causes fat-storage and metabolic sluggishness.

A balance of essential fatty acids and a balance of macro-nutrients (ratio of fat to protein to carbohydrate) is a key to optimal health.

In the wake of all the negative press about fats, in the mid 1990's several researchers began teaching and publishing popular books on how fats are the key to energy and health and play a major role in both weight issues and optimal health. They failed to address the reason that fats fell into disfavor with the pop nutritionists. The rampant confusion regarding fats in nutrition is spawned by the post-Industrial Revolution use of man-made and man-altered fats – more specifically the chemical processing of vegetable oil and the partial-hydrogenation of oil.

As you might expect, we need to stop the world and get off. People are being fed completely erroneous information by the media, spawned from the researchers, doctors, nutritionists and dietitians who either cannot see the whole picture or have a hidden agenda for financial profit. More than the example of the blind men and the elephant, information on fats is a clear example of the blind leading the blind.

Here's what Dr. Russell Smith, an expert on chronic heart disease says, "The relevant literature is permeated with fraudulent material that is designed to convert negative evidence into positive evidence with respect to the lipid [fat] hypothesis. That fraud is relatively easy to detect." Keep in mind that what Dr. Smith is calling "fraud" is what has shaped the information that the public understands about fat.

For example, we are told that cholesterol is bad, yet it is so important to the body that the body has two ways to get it to the cells because, without it, we would die. We are told that low-density lipid (LDL) cholesterol is the "bad" kind of fat, yet it is the LDL cholesterol that transports the beneficial essential fatty acid, linoleic acid, to the cells for the regulation of life processes.

Here's what the famous heart surgeon, Dr. Michael DeBakey, M.D., says. "An analysis of cholesterol values ... in 1700 patients with atherosclerotic disease revealed no definite correlation between serum cholesterol levels and the nature and extent of atherosclerotic disease." Along the same vein, the renowned researcher, Dr. George Mann, M.D., states, "The diet-heart hypothesis has been repeatedly shown to be wrong, and yet, for complicated reasons of pride, profit and prejudice, the hypothesis continues to be exploited by scientists, fund-raising enterprises, food companies, and even governmental agencies. The public is being deceived by the greatest health scam of the century."

Facts About Fats: "The fats and oils story may well be the greatest scandal of ignorance, disinformation, and greed in the entire history of food production."
- John Finnegan

Cholesterol is not the problem and is not the culprit in cardiovascular disease. But since this topic is not completely germane to our discussion of fat-burning, the cholesterol myth-busting story is in the *Eating Energy* book in case you want to learn more. The witch-hunt mentality regarding fats makes people point the finger at a particular fat and brand it "bad", when the crux of the problem is only one or both of the following two factors:

- the imbalance of fatty acids in the diet, and/or
- the commercial processing of fat.

A Nutrient Called Vitamin F – What Are Fats?

Fats are a macro-nutrient food substance found in seeds, vegetables, and other food sources of plant and animal origin, including meat, fish, dairy, and eggs. The term "fat" refers to the whole area of chemistry called *"fatty acids."* When the term "oil" is used, it refers to the fats that are liquid at room temperature. Fats and oils are in the nutritional category of "lipids," which includes all fat forms. Fats and oils are divided into categories according to their molecular structure and each different fatty acid performs vital functions in the body's life processes.

It would take quite a few pages to lay out the foundation of fatty acid chemistry. In fact, when I originally wrote it for this book, the pages numbered 30. Ultimately, this fascinating and critically-important knowledge is not so fascinating to the person who simply wants to know what to do to lose weight and improve health. Therefore, I will save the biochemistry lessons for the *Eating Energy* forum. Here, I will simply present the overview, the key essentials, of how you can virtually rebuild your health and reshape your body with the ShiftRight concept of bringing the beautiful and good fats into your diet and decreasing or eliminating the ugly, destructive fats.

In Praise of Fats

Currently, many fatty acids have been identified that support the human body. The number of fatty acids will undoubtedly increase as fat research continues. Here are few fatty-acid facts to improve the status of fats in our minds:

- Fat increases the metabolic rate, allowing more fat to be burned. You must eat fat to lose fat.

- Fats protect the body from protein catabolism (using tissue protein for energy).
- Fats allow the body to access protein better for muscle building.
- Fats allow your white blood cells to respond quicker to infections, and thus speed the healing process.
- Fats lubricate joints and keep the skin heathy.
- Fats help the metabolic rate, also called the oxidation rate, to be optimal. In fact, oils render more than twice as much energy as proteins and carbohydrates.
- Fats contribute to athletic stamina in two ways. Since fats are absorbed and processed slowly in the body, they provide a steady energy supply. This is important for the athlete because it is fat that the muscles burn for stamina. Also, fats allow for better combustion of glucose.
- Fats help get lactic acid out of the muscles, thus helping prevent soreness after exercise.
- Fats are a rich source of acetate, which prevents cellular exhaustion caused by the combustion of carbohydrates. For this reason, avocado (a food rich in oil) helps hypoglycemic people control and sustain the combustion of blood sugar and not have energy slumps.
- The mineral phosphorus cannot be absorbed through the intestinal wall, or be eliminated by the kidneys, without the use of oils. The reason for this is that phosphorus moves into and out of circulation as phospholipids, or in an oil-based form.
- Fatty acids are the major component of the cell membranes as well as inner cell membranes. (Fatty acids are akin to the wood, bricks, and stucco of a house as well as the sheet-rock of the walls inside the house.)

- Fats are the basis for hormones, including Human Growth Hormone (HGH) and testosterone.
- Essential Fatty Acids (EFA's) are vitally important for the thyroid and adrenal glands (our energy glands), the nerve sheath, the hair, skin and mucous membranes.
- EFA's play an important role in balancing cholesterol, blood clotting, proper blood pressure, glandular function and arterial flexibility.

ShiftRight With Fats Applying The Eating Energy 12 Optimal Nutrition Factors

By now, you have the general idea of a major cause of disease as well as why people have gained and stored so much fat-weight. It is the processing and altering of our food that has rendered unhealthy products. The post-Industrial Revolution processing and altering of fats in our diets has caused and is causing untold grief. Very simply, the ugly fats are killing us. Here, I'll briefly show you how to remedy this situation.

As you read these ShiftRight suggestions, you will understand the reason for the designation of fats as the beautiful, the good, the ugly. A simple shift from ugly fats to the use of beautiful and good fats will improve health and longevity dramatically. Let's put this theory to the test of the 12 Optimal Nutrition Factors.

1. **Quality.** The highest quality fats are the "beautiful" essential fatty acids in raw vegetables and seeds. The valuable oils in fish (EPA and DHA), while not *essential* oils, are so deficient in many people's diets that they too win the "beautiful" rating. Also, the "good" oils from olives and

other oil-rich vegetables and legumes are necessary and of excellent value, if they are consumed in their natural form. Once processing starts, the health benefits of the oil becomes compromised. The cheap, processed, heat-altered, hydrogenated, and partially-hydrogenated "ugly" oils are of unacceptable quality. For more specifics, see the sections of text about Beautiful Fats, Good Fats and Ugly Fats later in this chapter.

2. **Digestion.** The high quality "beautiful" and "good" fats contain enzymes and synergists that assist their digestion. When used properly, the body is well-adapted to digest them. The "ugly" oils are dead and warped. They tax the body's enzymes and detoxification processes to eliminate them.

3. **Assimilation/Humanization.** The "beautiful" and "good" oils assimilate well and are easily humanized and used by the body. The "ugly" processed fats deplete the body of its essential fatty acids and interfere with the body's life-processes.

4. **Bio-Availability (Low Stress).** The high-quality fats readily contribute to the body and move with ease into a position to provide energy and cell structure. The unacceptable ugly fats stress the liver and the body's free use of essential fatty acids.

5. **Balance of Macro-nutrient.** Fat is a macro-nutrient that should be balanced in the diet in two ways. First, the amount of fat should balance with the amount protein and carbohydrate. Second, fats can and should be balanced with the other types of fat in the diet as we see in the Natural fats in vegetables, seeds, olives, and fish for a variety of metabolic activities. The ugly (partially-hydrogenated trans-fats) are distorted creatures. These concepts are explained further in several sections of text later in this chapter.

6. **Complete, balanced Micro-Nutrients.** The "beautiful" and "good" oil foods contain all their natural vitamins, minerals, and nutrient synergists. The ugly fats are stripped of their vitamins, minerals, and synergists; also, their shape becomes unnatural, grotesque.

7. **Enzymes.** A whole, raw food contains inherent enzymes that aid in its digestion and assimilation. These are found in olives, nuts, seeds, avocados, sushi, ceviche, and raw vegetables. Cooking interferes with these enzymes and creates the need for additional digestive resources from the body. [The addition of raw vegetables helps in digestion.]

8. **pH (acid/alkaline balance).** The high quality fats fulfill their role as acids in body metabolism. The low quality fats confuse the metabolism with poor facsimiles of fatty acids and contribute to excessive junk acid in the body. Fatty acids carry the yang spark of vitality (an acid pH) and impart vital energy to the body in the presence of the alkaline reserve (minerals provided by vegetables).

9. **Fiber.** The high quality fats in vegetables and seeds are accompanied by natural fiber that controls their rate of absorption. Fiber has been removed from refined, processed, bleached, heated, sanitized, hydrogenated and partially-hydrogenated fats.

10. **Water content.** Fats are not water-soluble by their nature. They are made water-soluble by digestion and protein. Many natural fatty foods such as vegetables and fish also contain inherent water and protein (amino acids).

11. **Detoxification.** The liver uses beautiful and good fats for detoxification. Ugly fats contribute to the toxic burden of

the body both by their altered structure and by the pesticides that accompany them.

12. **Bio-energy.** Beautiful and good fats contain the energy of the sun in their molecules and are virtually a spark of life. They contribute to and support the body's energy, both biochemically and bio-energetically and recharge the body's life energies. The dead, heat and chemically-altered fats do not contribute to the life force as this essential element has been completely destroyed. Instead, they rob precious vitality from the cells.

The Beautiful Fats

The liver synthesizes all but two of the many beneficial fatty acids. The "Beautiful" Essential Fatty Acids (Alpha Linolenic-omega-3, and Linoleic-omega-6) come from nature in an unprocessed state. They are powerhouses of stored energy. These two important fatty acids have been designated as *Essential Fatty Acids (EFA's)*, meaning that *we must have a dietary intake of them.* EFA's, along with their natural synergists (enzymes, nutrients, other fatty acids,) bring energy, nutrients, health, and stamina by directly supporting the body's entire fatty acid metabolism. EFA's are the fats that balance the cells' micro-hormones, called "eicosanoids," and control the body's hormonal responses that control key areas of health including weight loss, blood pressure, and the immune system. EFA benefits include the following. They:

- keep arteries soft and pliable
- maintain proper blood pressure
- prevent blood clots

- lower cholesterol production in the liver, regulating cholesterol and triglycerides
- prevent cell proliferation (cancer)
- improve the immune response (For every "-itis" there is a fatty acid involved in the immune response)
- decrease inflammation
- decrease pain transmission
- reduce histamine response (Help decrease allergies)
- control release of lymphokines (Reduce allergies)
- prevent auto-immune diseases
- support cell membrane structures without which the cells become subject to infections, die, fail metabolically and become allergy-prone
- provide essential support for neurological function, (brain, adrenals, eyes)
- increase the body's ability to absorb oxygen for energy
- reduce the time for fatigued muscles to recover
- increase metabolic activities
- regulate sodium and water retention.

You can see that essential fatty acids hold the key to the major health concerns facing humanity today – heart and cardiovascular disease, cancer, and the immune system (allergies, diseases.) With something this important, we certainly do not want a low fat diet. We will choke off our supply of critically important nutrients and their ability to be our strong allies. We must have a "right fat" diet that includes the "beautiful" fats.

Now you've probably been told more than you ever wanted to know about fat chemistry, so I hope you endured it all. We've only discussed the very tip of this subject. At least now I hope you have an appreciation for the power of fats and their many benefits. Now, let's focus on what all this really means.

If the essential fatty acids control the major health and disease processes in our bodies, *what controls the fatty acids?* Would you believe — the balance of macro-nutrients (protein and carbohydrate) controls the fatty acids because of the body's hormonal response to food. This is based on the opposing hormones insulin and glucagon. Ah, we've been here before!

The following table shows the foods that contain both EFA's or the beneficial marine lipids — EPA/DHA — and, thus, provide a superior level of nutrition.

The terrific, Beautiful Fats have both essential fatty acids, or have especially beneficial forms of fatty acids that bring positive health benefits.

- Flaxseed oil (processed with care, not linseed oil)
- Hemp seed oil (legal issues have kept this valuable oil out of circulation)
- Pumpkin Seed and Pumpkin seed oil
- Walnuts and Walnut oil
- Seaweed (Kelp, Dulse, Nori, etc.)
- Dark green vegetables (broccoli, kale, spinach, parsley, etc.)

The following "beautiful" oils contain special fatty acids that support health by providing specific beneficial fats that clean the arteries and balance the hormones:

- Fish Oils (EPA, DHA) from ocean-run salmon, sardines, mackerel, trout, eel and in smaller amounts in clams, oysters, scallops, squid, shrimp, lobster, muscles, crab, conch
- Evening Primrose Oil [a rich source of a valuable oil called gamma linolenic acid (GLA)] primes the hormone pathway that fights disease.

The fats listed in the previous table are the "super-beneficial" fats. There are still many more fats that are beneficial in human nutrition. They are listed as the "Good Fats" to follow.

The Good Fats

The "good fats" can contain one rather than both of the essential fats, or other beneficial or non-detrimental fats such as oleic acid (omega-9). These fats are the ones that work for the body in its myriad functions, particularly for energy and caloric heat. Good fats are associated with the fat-soluble vitamins such as Vitamins A, D, E, and K. In correct amounts, the "good" fats can occur in Nature in three forms: saturated, polyunsaturated, and monounsaturated, which are designations of their molecular structure. These various fats help with the body's biochemistry.

The Good Fats have a place in our diets along with the beautiful fats.

- Almonds and almond oil
- Avocado
- Balanced butter (organic, raw milk butter with added flaxseed and grapeseed oil, vitamin E and lecithin. Best used in a diet low in saturated fat.)
- Butter (Organic, raw milk. Contains very short chain fatty acids that provide anti-tumor effects. Contains conjugated linoleic acid, which has anti-cancer properties.)
- Grapeseed Oil
- Macadamia nuts
- Nuts (Some nuts were singled out as particularly beneficial, either in this list or in the Beautiful Fats list, and others include brazil, cashew, filbert, pecans, pine nuts, etc.)
- Olives and extra virgin olive oil (expeller-pressed or cold-processed)
- Raw milk cheeses (Feta, Cottage Cheese)

(continued on next page)

(Good Fats – continued from previous page)

- Seeds (Some seeds were singled out as particularly beneficial, either in this list or in the Beautiful Fats list. Others include sunflower, squash, chia, and others.)
- Safflower oil, high oleic
- Sesame seeds and sesame oil, Tahini
- Sunflower oil, high oleic
- Unrefined Coconut Oil (Contains medium chain fatty acids with anti-fungal properties.)
- Soy bean oil (from non-hybridized soy beans. The hybridized beans have reduced linolenic acid content.)

The Ugly Fats

The ugly fats are those that have been made rancid by heat, light, or oxygen. They are the ones that have been processed, hydrogenated, and, even worse – *partially-hydrogenated.* They include both the altered vegetable mono and polyunsaturated fats as well as the altered animal and vegetable saturated fats. [Note: the body has a requirement for saturated fat, it's the *altered* saturated fats, along with other *altered* fats, that cause the problems with the cardiovascular system.] Ugly fats are the culprits – the ones that destroy the heart, the arteries, and cause cancer. During commercial processing of fats, the heat and partial-hydrogenation of fats, the molecules are altered or straightened out. These molecules, called *trans fatty acids*, cause terrible damage to people's health.

Natural Law: Foods from Nature, unchanged, serve human health and bring prosperity. Alterations of Nature's design bring sub-optimal nutrition and disease.

Normal fatty acids are horseshoe-shaped structures, which is the shape of the Greak letter "omega" – hence the use of that word in fatty acid chemistry. In this shape, fatty acids can provide an interlocking structure to cell walls and membranes. When high heat and artificial hydrogenation creates *trans form* fatty acids, the molecules lose their horseshoe shape and become more straight. Although the body attempts to burn these trans fats, some get incorporated into the cell membranes where they become a weak link because they no longer fit the interlocking pattern. They leave a gap for viruses and bacteria to invade. They can also create a weak structure that can be susceptible to abnormal cellular processes – cancer. The body is capable of dealing with some of the *trans* fatty acids. It can recognize the twisted, warped, and malformed molecules and destroy them. Unfortunately, many people eat more *trans*-fat than the body can possibly handle. Some researchers suspect this is a possible reason that cancer has increased proportionally with the use of partially-hydrogenated fat.

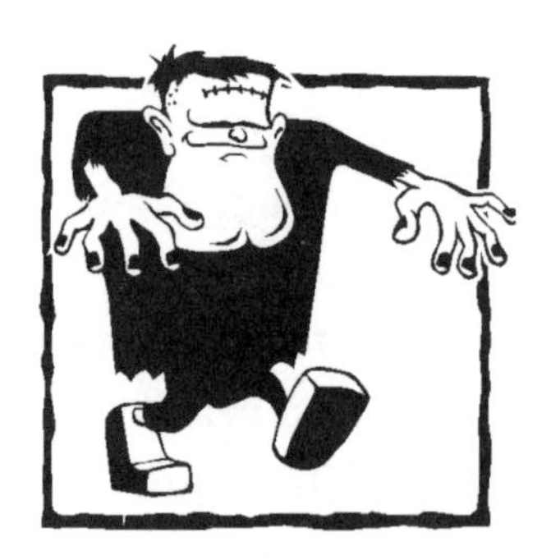

The Health Risks of Using Trans Fatty Acids and Rancid Oils

Trans fatty acids are strongly linked with cancer, atherosclerosis, and chronic-degenerative disease. The major sources of *trans* fatty acids are margarine, shortening, French-fries, candy, microwave popcorn, and bakery products. In the body, they generate free-radical molecules that destroy cells and interact with cholesterol to form plaque that damages the arteries. *Trans* fatty acids can increase blood cholesterol by 20% and increase triglycerides by 50%.

A warning about detrimental oils is also in order. Many nutritionists know that oils can be the most damaging food substance if used improperly as in chips, candy, and fried food. In fact, if oils are rancid, they are quite poisonous. For this reason, many nutritionists believe that the fast food industry is a leader in destroying human health. Three of the very real factors connecting oil to cancer are the **rancidity, processing** and **heating** of the oil. Here is a brief discussion of dangerous rancid oils; again, much has been omitted for the sake of brevity.

The oils designated "partially-hydrogenated," as well as the highly processed oils sold in grocery stores are a major factor in cardiovascular disease. These products of the Industrial Revolution, along with the homogenization of milk, put detrimental fats into the body. When these fats are oxidized, they cause vast damage. This information is really a tangent to our understanding of how to manage fats in our diets (especially to the end of losing excessive stored fat) but it is an important topic – one that may save your life and the lives of family members and others. Thus, I recommend the book *Eating Energy* if you are interested in reading more.

It's not fats in your diet that cause health concerns. It's the processed, partially-hydrogenated oils called trans-fats that are destroying health.

Paralleling the rise in the use of processed, commercial vegetable oils was a rise in cardiovascular disease, cancer, multiple sclerosis, diabetes, and liver degenerative diseases. Even the phenomenal advances and technologies of modern medicine could not stem the damaging effects of processed oil. Since the turn of the century, cardiovascular disease has increased 390%. Cancer has increased 635%. Many researchers think refined vegetable oil is the greatest killer in the world.

What can you do?

- First, throw out the shortening and processed vegetable oils.
- Buy organically grown, properly processed grapeseed oil, flaxseed oil, extra-virgin olive oil, or sesame oil, available at many

health food stores. Essential fatty acids as found in flaxseed oil and grapeseed oil actually help the body overcome the effects of *trans*-fatty acids.

- Anti-oxidant nutrients such as selenium; vitamins A, C, E; pycnogenol, alpha lipoic acid, and grapeseed extract may also help reduce the damage of *trans*-fats.
- Supplement with omega 3 capsules.

All we need to do is shift our diets right from the ugly partially-hydrogenated oils to the beautiful essential fatty acids (or, for a lesser effect, to the good fatty acids,) and a major change will occur in our body's ability to maintain optimal health.

Avoid These "Ugly" Fats

- Partially-hydrogenated oils (in candy, chips, shortening, commercial bakery goods)
- Margarine (major source of *trans* fatty acids)
- Lard, heated (excessive saturated fat)
- Hydrogenated oils (heat altered, dead)
- Processed oils (heat altered, manipulated, changed)
- Shortening (major source of *trans* fatty acids)
- Canola Oil (genetically altered, used to make mustard gas)
- Corn Oil (highly processed, but good inside the corn kernel)
- Soy Oil (highly processed, but good inside the bean)
- Cotton Seed Oil (often contains pesticides)

What Is The Correct Daily Amount Of Fat?

The body's nutrient requirement of beneficial (beautiful and good) fats is generally between one and two tablespoons a day. Virtually everyone is deficient in essential fatty acids, especially the essential fat, linolenic acid. Few people realize that the body has a nutritional requirement for essential fatty acids, just like it does for other vitamins and nutrients. Fats, like batteries, are storehouses of energy and are used for energy metabolism, glandular integrity, skin, heart function and the immune system.

For weight-loss purposes, nutritionists recommend that fats should comprise between 20 and 35 percent of the daily caloric intake. Generally, this is more than people with a "low-fat" mentality are currently consuming. In your dietary recommendation *for The Weight Is Over* program, your fat requirement will be addressed automatically by the high-quality protein and vegetable foods along with the other macro-nutrients.

Your correct amount of fat is dependent on several factors including:

- muscle mass,
- quality of the fat,
- balance of fatty acids in your diet,
- balance with the other macro-nutrients.

So you can see that our mission is to ShiftRight and get it right. That's all. *The Weight Is Over* will help you with an instant solution to very complex issues, just by incorporating the summary advice in this chapter.

Most people have a deficiency of essential fatty acids and overload of detrimental fats because they neglect the "beautiful" fats and use the "ugly". As we might predict, under such circumstances, health becomes ugly. Although fats are a critically important nutrient, misused oils are the most potentially dangerous food substances we eat – causing cancer, hardened arteries, high blood pressure and heart attacks.

The Eating Energy 50:50 - A Balance of Essential Fatty Acids

The brain is mostly made of fat. Besides bringing a whole new meaning to the term "lard-brain," the brain is a 50:50 balance between the two essential fatty – the beautiful fats. It is also rich in cholesterol. Thus, we find that Nature's choice for the function of the body's key organ is equal parts of both essential fats.

Actually, a delicate check-and-balance system exists between the two essential fats. The production of all eicosanoids for a balanced body chemistry depends on a balance of essential fatty acids. Too much or too little of either one or the other can result in the body leaning too far from the optimal balance. Many of the leading fatty acid researchers recommend a 50:50 balance of essential fatty acids.

Many nutritionists like to capitalize on omega-3 oils (such as flaxseed and fish oils) dietarily because the American diet leans heavily into omega-6, due to the preponderance of vegetable oils. In 1991, the *American Journal of Clinical Nutrition* reported,

> *"Americans consume far too much of one kind of EFA (omega-6 found in most polyunsaturated vegetable oils), but not enough of another kind of EFA (omega-3 found in fish, fish oils, eggs from properly raised chickens, dark green vegetables, herbs such as purslane, and oils from certain seeds such as flaxseed and chia, nuts such as walnuts and, in small amounts, in all whole grains)."*

What Does a Deficiency of Fats Cause?

When people do not have a sufficient supply of essential fatty acids, many of the body's metabolic processes are retarded or stop completely. The super-powerful micro-hormones, eicosanoids, which initiate the fat-burning processes, depend upon a balance of essential fatty acids to be able to perform their critical regulatory roles that occur in a microsecond. Thus, fats are absolutely essential ingredient in losing weight. Symptoms of a diet deficient in essential fat include:

- Acne
- Allergies
- Amenorrhea
- Atherosclerosis
- Diarrhea, chronic
- Eczema
- Fatigue
- Gall stones
- Hair loss
- Healing process slow
- Hormonal imbalance
- Immune system weakness
- Marasmus (failure to thrive)
- Menopausal symptoms (hot flashes)
- Menstrual problems
- Nail weakness
- Nerve weakness
- Platelet adhesions (sticky blood)
- Prostate, enlarged
- Reproductive organ dysfunction
- Skin problems, dry
- Stamina, poor
- Varicose veins
- Wrinkled skin

What Does An Excess of Fats Cause?

If too many of the beneficial fats are included in the diet (highly unlikely), a person becomes sluggish. When too many detrimental fats are consumed, the likelihood of heart disease, cancer, hypoglycemia, allergies, obesity, food sensitivities, sluggish liver, gall stones and endocrine gland dysfunction is greatly increased. Symptoms of too many ugly fats and the imbalance of fats in the diet include:

- Acne
- Bad breath
- Bloating
- Body odor, strong
- Cardiovascular disease
- Cholesterol problems
- Chronic, degenerative diseases
- Constipation

- Dysmenorrhea
- Fatigue 2 hrs. after eating
- Gall stones
- Gas
- Heart disease
- Menopausal symptoms
- Mood swings
- Oily skin
- Prostate problems
- Tension
- Yellow, white, or gray stool
- Water retention

Fats are fabulous nutrients when used the way that Nature intended. The more we adopt the natural use of fats, the less we have to worry about ugly fats hurting our health. With a proper dietary focus, we earn back the right to enjoy butter and eggs, basic natural foods – at least before commercialization. Organize your pantry and kitchen to ShiftRight back into a full and varied use of Nature's foods known as *beneficial* and *good* fats. Protect yourself from the damage of the *ugly* fats. Better health and better weight is only a plate away!

CHAPTER ELEVEN

Fats: Health and Fat Loss Tips

Eating By Association

Eating carbohydrates and snack foods that contain ugly, partially-hydrogenated fats often occurs habitually with certain activities (for example, eating popcorn at the movies or crunching on chips and slurping a soda when watching your favorite TV show). One patient reported to me, "I gained 20 pounds watching Ally McBeal lose weight on TV!" The combination of eating refined carbohydrate, eating ugly fat foods, and the activity form an *engram* (an association) in the brain. This association makes it more difficult to break the habit of eating detrimental foods when that activity is being done.

"Vegging out" with the TV ought to mean snacking on crispy, raw vegetables.

During your fat-loss program, you may need to break that association in order to break free of the snack food-addiction pattern. If you associate watching TV with eating snacks, you may need to give up TV (heaven forbid!) for a while, or you may be successful in substituting something else in the snack's place. For example, I consulted with a man who simply drank "shots" of bottled water while watching football on TV. The tiny portions of water somehow tasted different and kept him engaged in something new. It worked. It was a terrific substitution for what was usually two pints of ice cream.

If you need to abandon an activity because it is your Waterloo and causes you to revert to old habits, take on a new project.

Tackle a home improvement, a new hobby, clean out the garage instead of "vegging out" with TV. Start a garden. Meet with friends to bike around the lake – whatever it takes.

Quick Guide: Handle Oils With Care!

Since the misuse of oils can cause so many health problems, we need to take a look at how to work with oils to obtain the benefits without the liabilities. The following are some suggestions for proper, healthful use of oils.

- Flaxseed oil is wonderful for cold, supplemental use. Don't cook it! Grapeseed oil and sesame oil (unrefined) are also good for salads because of their anti-rancid factors. Extra virgin olive oil, rich in oleic acid, offers protection to the heart by reducing the low density lipoprotein (LDL cholesterol is often called "bad cholesterol"), while leaving the high density lipoproteins (HDL is often called "good cholesterol").
- Use sesame oil with other oils. It prevents rancidity inside the body.
- Use cooking oils very sparingly.
- Use grapeseed or peanut oil for cooking. They have high flash points and thus do not turn toxic as quickly as other oils. Never save heated oil and never reuse heated oil.
- Use extra virgin olive oil to obtain monounsaturated acids. Olive oil is known to help prevent gallstones if used once a week. It also has anti-candida (fungus) properties and anti-LDL-cholesterol factors.
- The very best sources of oil are those locked inside the cells of a plant. Next best are cold-processed flax seed oil, grapeseed oil and extra virgin olive oil.

- Expeller-pressed oils are preferred. "Cold pressed" is a meaningless term since the oil is pressed cold, but heated when it is not being pressed. The term is simply a marketing hoax. "Cold-processed" is a more meaningful term because the oil's temperature is kept low. However, the processing may involve skelly oil (hexane) as a solvent. Expeller-pressed oils are consistently high quality. To insure high quality, buy oils from the health food store, but even then, check the oil's quality since many "health food" oils are "cold pressed" to temperatures of 140-180 degrees F.
- Store oil in the refrigerator in dark colored bottles or cans. More companies provide this consideration these days. Do not expose oil to heat or light. Do not shake the bottle because this contributes to oxidation.
- Wipe the rim of the bottle and cap off after each use. Avoid rancidity.
- Never choose fried foods. Avoid them. They're not fit to eat.
- Avoid wheat germ oil pearls, seed meals, dry lecithin or commercial wheat germ. They are usually rancid.
- Cottonseed oil usually contains pesticides.
- Use natural vitamin E from 100% vegetable sources as a protective dietary supplement when using oils.
- Avoid margarine and any oil that stays solid at room temperature (shortening). These partially-hydrogenated oils are unnatural and are linked with cancer. Instead, use organic butter sparingly. Tahini can be a good butter substitute. Olive oil is a good butter substitute and is featured in top Italian restaurants for dipping bread.
- When stir-frying, heat the skillet or wok to a low temperature first, (250 degrees F) then add two Tbs. water rather

than oil. Many fine cooks simply toss the vegetables in a little oil and add them to the wok with a little water. This minimizes the oxidation of both the oil and the vegetables.

- Eggs can be poached without oil in a skillet of water and a little vinegar.

CHAPTER TWELVE

Carbohydrates' Role In Fat-Burning and Health

You are not a dough-boy!
- Dr. A. S. Wheelwright

What Is A Carbohydrate?

Most people think carbohydrates mean starchy food. Actually, carbohydrates include all starches and sugars. So carbohydrates include alcohol (beer, wine, whiskey), all vegetables, grains (bread, spaghetti, chips, rice, cereals), fruit, potatoes, candy and sugar-desserts (pie, cake, ice cream). What allows for such a wide range? It's simply the many variations on the theme of carbohydrate molecules. Despite the many variations, there are two primary categories of carbohydrates – simple sugars and complex carbohydrates, plus one "new" category that's been added in the past 125 years, *processed, refined carbohydrates.*

- **Simple sugars**, such as those found in fruit, many vegetables, and milk require little digestion and enter the blood stream readily.
- **Complex carbohydrates** require the most digestive processing and provide the body the most control over their conversion to glucose – the body's energy fuel. Many complex carbohydrates are found in vegetables and whole grains.
- There is a deadly, third category of carbohydrates that emerged as the Industrial Revolution began. It's the **processed, refined carbohydrates** as found in "refined" sugar, "refined" flour pastas, instant mashed potatoes, rice cakes,

corn flakes, white bread, chips, cookies, pastries, candy, and desserts. These products have an elevated glycemic index due to the heating and processing as well as a lowered nutritional value. The glycemic index is a measurement of how fast a food delivers glucose to the bloodstream.

The Glycemic Index

This brings us to the subject of the glycemic index of foods. "Glycemic" refers to how quickly a sugar is processed into glucose. There are several studies on how quickly starch and sugars are broken down and stimulate the pancreas to secrete insulin in response to them. Many nutritionists use the glycemic index tables, as a general, ballpark guide to carbohydrates to determine what constitutes a balanced meal.

Gee, he's sweet!
I wonder what his
glycemic index is?

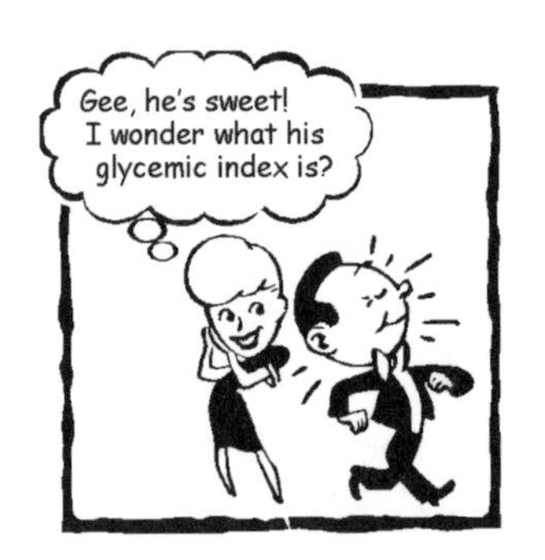

There are several, individually-defined factors that modify the glycemic effect of carbohydrates. Each person has his/her own tolerance of glucose that is based on genetics and the amount of wear and tear (sugar abuse) he/she has experienced. Further, a person who has protein and fat early in the day has more stability in their hormonal response to glucose because they have "buffers" to the uninhibited expression of glucose metabolism. Also, keep in mind that the total carbohydrate content of a food can include fiber, which is not metabolically active in that it does not convert to sugar, and actually serves to control the rate of sugar induction into the blood stream.

The general idea of a glycemic index provides some interesting insights to the effects of carbohydrates on the body. If a person is carbohydrate sensitive as in hypoglycemia, the foods with a high glycemic index can more easily cause an overreaction by the pancreas to produce insulin, whereas foods lower in the glycemic index are more gentle and less damaging. So high glycemic-index foods have more stressful levels of sugar than low glycemic-index foods. We include the glycemic index of a carbohydrate as one factor in determining its role in nutrition. In the *Eating Energy* 12 Optimal Nutrition Factors, it fits into the Macro-Nutrient Balance category. A quick-reference list is provided in "Appendix A: Glycemic Index." Become familiar with that information as it will alert you to potentially damaging foods and help you focus on those that support health and your efforts to burn fat.

Here's an example. The glycemic index of fructose, the simple sugar in an apple is 26. The glycemic index of white bread is 100, the same as pure glucose. Thus, a natural apple is much less aggravating to the carbohydrate metabolism than hybridized, processed wheat (white bread.) Here we see that a natural carbohydrate food is fine, while a processed, refined carbohydrate food is potentially damaging.

People often ask, "Does a fruit have too much sugar? Should I avoid fruit?" A fruit is a natural food that contains some simple sugars in the form of fructose. Fruit also contains complex sugars and cellulose that allow a more steady processing of the sugars. A fruit is mostly water by volume and a fine food when used the *Eating Energy* way — generally eaten by themselves for a refreshing afternoon or evening snack.

Although natural, simple carbohydrates are processed quickly in the body, they do not inflict the damage that refined sugars do. A fruit is only 15% simple carbohydrates (sugars), whereas a refined grain such as pasta can be 75% simple carbohydrates.

What Is The Role Of carbohydrates In The Body?

Carbohydrates are generally known to serve four purposes:

- energy metabolism,
- protein conservation,
- fiber, and
- miscellaneous specialized functions such as the assimilation of calcium, making compounds for genetic coding, and other ways the body might tear carbohydrates down for their basic elements – carbon, hydrogen, oxygen.

Carbohydrates are the basis of our cellular fuel system. They are processed into glucose, the sugar our cells use for biochemical energy. The brain and nervous system use glucose as high-energy fuel for their high-energy functions. These tissues claim an immediate-need priority for glucose. This priority contributes to the body's strong desire for carbohydrates and sugar that plagues people as part of their craving for sweets.

Carbohydrate excesses may have caused a person to become obese, but complex carbohydrates (vegetables) are needed to properly lose fat-weight.

A health perspective on carbohydrate storage is similar to that of gasoline storage for your car. It's great to have a full tank, ready to burn and propel the car wherever you want to go. It's not so great to have excess gasoline in the trunk, on the seat next to you, and sloshing three inches deep on the floor.

Carbohydrates are needed, even for weight loss. Carbohydrates conserve the use of vital proteins. They spare the body's precious nucleo-proteins from being burned for energy. Thus, the right amount of carbohydrate protects the body's lean muscle mass, and, with the right amount of protein in the diet, the body will access fat (rather than the muscles) for energy. A diet without carbohydrates will result in ketosis, the converting of fat and protein (muscles) into glucose. This can cause rapid weight loss, but it also causes undesirable side effects including brain fog, fatigue, mood swings, forgetfulness, sluggishness and loss of muscle. In such an imbalanced state, the fat cells are primed to regain their lost molecular gold. Thus, when a person begins eating carbohydrates again, the weight re-gain can be horrendous. The Urk genes fight for survival and the person is prone to massive weight gain.

Dietary/Metabolic Equation:

Right carbohydrates

+

Right fats

+

Right proteins

The body burns fat for energy rather than the muscle-protein or glucose alone.

How Do I ShiftRight With Carbohydrates Into The Fat-Burning Dimension?

To ShiftRight into the optimal use of carbohydrates, we must generally do four things:

1. Reduce and/or eliminate refined sugar.
2. Reduce and/or eliminate processed carbohydrates (refined grains: breads, cereals.)

3. Eat more high quality carbohydrates, specifically vegetables and fruit.
4. Balance carbohydrate intake with high quality proteins and fats.

Carbohydrate foods exist on a continuum. On the left side we have the very detrimental carbohydrates. These include refined sugar, processed starchy foods, and alcohol, as well as hybridized, processed high-glycemic grains. Now, ShiftRight. On the right side, we have Nature's best, the vegetables. By vegetables I mean fresh green, red, white, yellow, purple, or orange vegetables, the kind that grow in the garden, often called "pot-herbs." People today often call a potato a "vegetable" which is factually true, but from our fat-weight loss perspective a potato is a starch, as are rice and grains. Starches can be fine foods when used as whole foods (unrefined, unprocessed) and balanced with other vegetables and macro-nutrients.

Whole grains, such as amaranth, spelt, red winter wheat, Indian corn, barley, whole grain rice, rye, quinoa, millet, and so forth will fall in the middle of the continuum. Between the grains and vegetables fall the fruits and carrots (along with other vegetables like beets and parsnips) which have a higher glycemic index than vegetables such as cabbage.

I once had a patient tell me, "I eat from all three food groups – a hamburger (protein, fat) and fries (French fried potatoes – carbohydrate). This is really the perfect example of the difference between the dietician or food chemist telling us that a hamburger and fries is a balanced meal vs the *Eating Energy* perspective of *quality* nutrition. Instead of the burger, how about a balanced meal of free-range chicken breast on an organically-grown garden salad with a flaxseed and extra virgin olive oil dressing? Run your nutritional calculator and apply the

12 Optimal Nutrition Factors. The burger and fries becomes a negative food (heat-altered saturated fat, growth hormone residues, antibiotic residues, empty calories in the refined bun, pesticides, rancid fats, partially-hydrogenated oil, low water content, empty starch, chemical additives.) Gulp!

How is the carbohydrate continuum derived? It comes from the 12 *Eating Energy* Optimal Nutrition Factors. This includes complexity of the food, digestibility, the fiber, the glycemic index, the availability of vitamins and minerals, the ability to impart vitality (electromagnetic energy), water content, the presence of pesticides and chemicals, and so forth.

Which Are The Ultimate Carbohydrate Foods for Human Nutrition?

Let's use our 12 questions, the *Eating Energy* Optimal Nutrition Factors, to look at carbohydrate foods to derive the best ones for human nutrition. Right now, we can separate the wheat from the chaff so to speak, and establish a list of carbohydrates that we want in our diets as well as a list of carbohydrates to avoid.

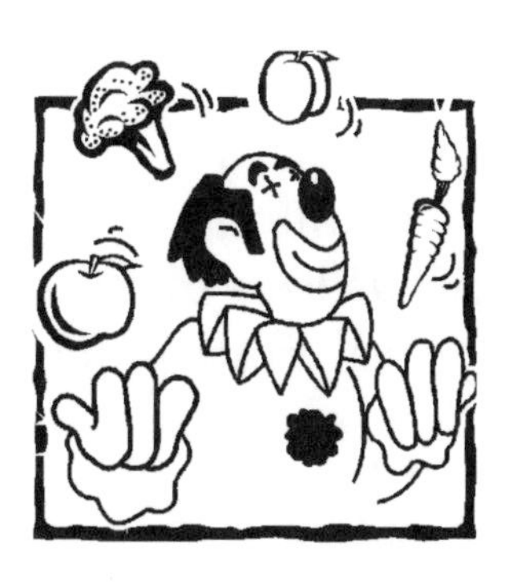

Every food has its pros and cons. One food, such as a potato, may be rich in fiber, but also be high in its glycemic index. The issue will then be how well the fiber modifies the absorption of sugar. Another food might be a great complex carbohydrate, but it also contains phytates – a chemical that inhibits the absorption of zinc, calcium, and magnesium – making it less than optimal on the assimilation question. We'll have to look at many factors to derive a list of optimal carbohydrates, and then rely on the variety principle to minimize any detrimental aspects and maximize the overall nutrition.

1. **Quality:** The highest quality carbohydrates are raw vegetables and fruit because, generally, they can be used as they come from nature, without processing. These whole foods are complete with enzymes, vitamins, minerals, water and fiber as nature intended. They do not surprise the liver and pancreas with excessive sugar or empty calories because they allow the body's natural enzyme processes to digest and assimilate the sugars gradually.

   Next, we find that some vegetables require light cooking before they are edible, such as peas, beans, green beans, lima beans, potato, yam, and so forth. The heat of cooking destroys the enzymes, so these foods will not receive an optimal grade for that reason, but the heat is needed to break down some of the tough cellulose, so the body can digest the food. Also, the heat may be used to break down antiproteolytic enzymes that block protein assimilation and thus render the food usable. Further, *New Scientist Magazine* reports a study that cooking certain vegetables (such as carrots, brussel sprouts, lima beans, green beans, black-eyed peas, and squash) increases the amount of carotenoid compounds that can fight cancer and protect against heart disease. Absorption of carotenoids from raw carrots is around 4%. Absorption of carotenoids from cooked carrots is around 20%.

Variety in the diet allows the body to capitalize on the best nutrition of many foods and minimize any undesirable effects.

   Next, but nowhere as superior as raw vegetables and fruit, would be primitive, whole grains such as spelt, buckwheat, amaranth, quinoa, oats, barley, and rye. As the grain goes higher up the glycemic index, the more hybridized it is, or the more processed it is, the less suitable it is for valuable human nutrition. The next lower level of grains would include rice, wheat, millet, and corn.

The Pro-Vita! Plan For Optimal Nutrition *established a dietary rule of having one cooked plus four raw vegetables with every meal. This rule is adopted intact in the* Eating Energy *plan.*

2. **Digestion:** Generally, raw vegetables such as salads digest well because they contain their own digestive enzymes. For some people, the digestion of raw vegetables causes problems because their weak digestive systems struggle to break down the complex starch and protein fibers. Such people need a program to build their digestive capabilities, so they can earn back the ability to eat raw vegetables. In naturopathic practice, nutritionists often approach this symptom with enzyme supplements.

   However, for people with trouble digesting raw vegetables, lightly steamed vegetables work well and are still superior to grain products. The heat of cooking will break down the vegetable's cellulose fibers and help the body assimilate the nucleic acids in the inner cell of the vegetable. It is unfortunate that cooking destroys some of the vitamins and all of the enzymes. That's why cooking must be light – just a light steaming, or a light stir-fry technique.

3. **Assimilation:** Once vegetables are properly digested, they assimilate very well. The water inherent in vegetables provides an escort service for easy assimilation. The fiber content helps with the proper assimilation of sugars and vegetable oils. Vegetables help with the assimilation of proteins and fats.

4. **Macro-Nutrient Balance:** Vegetables provide the optimal carbohydrate because they can easily be balanced with other foods that provide protein and essential fatty acids. Grains can also provide carbohydrate, but since they are cooked into starch, there can be some difficulty in combining grains with protein. For many people, a concentrated protein/concentrated starch combination (steak and potato) is not digested well, resulting in putrefaction of the protein in the bowel. Vegetables are the universal carbohydrate.

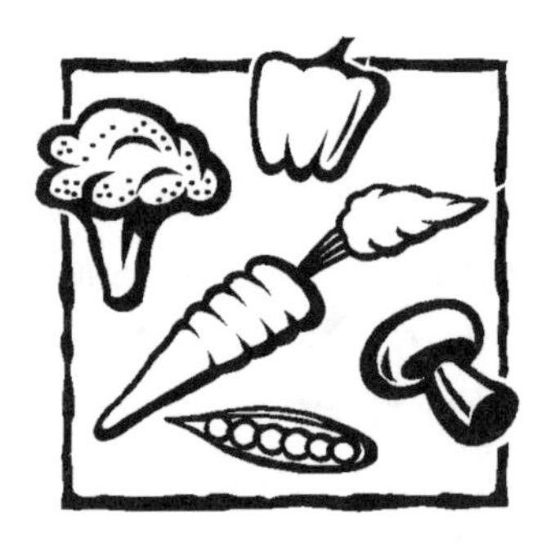

5. **Micro-Nutrient Balance:** Raw vegetables and fruit provide vitamins, minerals, and trace minerals, in Nature's ratios, plus other valuable phytonutrients such as anti-oxidants, lignins, isoflavones and carotenoid complexes. Organically-raised produce contains Nature's bounty of trace elements. It is far superior to grains, and processed foods as sources of micronutrients.

6. **Enzymes:** We've covered the fact that only raw foods (particularly vegetables and fruit) retain the enzymes necessary for their ease of digestion. These food-enzymes help preserve your interior enzyme reserve so your enzymes can perform other functions, such as cleaning up the bloodstream, protecting your arteries, keeping your vision acute, and helping your brain think. They also relieve the immune system from having to help digest food, so your immune cells can be better utilized in keeping you healthy. More on this in the *Eating Energy* book. You are as young as your enzymes!

7. **pH:** Raw and lightly cooked vegetables and fruit provide the body with the minerals to support the alkaline reserve, which is the basis for detoxification and health. Generally,

cooked grains also provide minerals, but they lean toward being acid-forming. Refined sugars disturb the acid/alkaline balance, causing acid reactions and a negative nutritional toll as the body must labor to buffer the acidic effects. To give further but brief explanation to this topic, the problem being addressed here is the current dietary shift to the left of the pH scale into the acid range, due to the eating of too many acid foods and not enough of the alkaline healers. For optimal health, we need a balance between the acids of protein and fatty acids and the alkaline foods, which are primarily vegetables.

8. **Fiber:** The best fibers are in raw vegetables and fruit. Cooked fibers in grains are helpful, but not the optimal highest quality. Tomatoes, apples and strawberries are known for their superior fiber. Because the Standard American Diet (SAD – and it really is) is now low in fiber due to the milling and processing of grains and avoidance of vegetables, many people take a fiber supplement such as apple pectin, cellulose, psyllium husks and so forth.

9. **Water content:** Raw vegetables and fruit excel in water content, which serves as a delivery system for their vitamins, minerals, and proteins. This water is also a valuable cleanser of cellular debris. The water in raw fruit and vegetables is filtered and organized by the phyto life form. It is optimal for human health.

10. **Bio-Availability:** *The lowest-stress carbohydrates are vegetables and fruit – especially raw ones.* Their nutrients are bio-available, non-heat-altered, and alive with enzymes, making them a truly perfect food and an excellent food to combine with other food groups for maximum assimilation of usable nutrients. The grains are often allergenic and can

have anti-proteolytic factors that inhibit protein digestion or phytates that inhibit mineral absorption.

11. **Detoxification:** Organically-grown vegetables and fruit contain no pesticides, additives, preservatives or hormones. Thus, they are low stress regarding toxicity level. As mentioned, the water content helps the body detoxify cellular wastes, making raw vegetables and fruits premier foods for health. If you can't always get organic vegetables, *The Pro-Vita! Plan For Optimal Nutrition* explains a soaking technique that help rid produce of pesticides, for those who are interested.

12. **Bio-energy:** The living nutrients in raw vegetables and fruit virtually sing with bio-magnetic energy as shown in Kirlian photography (a method of capturing essential energy on film.) When picked at the peak of vine-, tree-, or plant-ripeness, the full focus of the plant's vitality is present. The living enzymes are powerhouses of vital energy, making these foods true to "life begets life." Raw vegetables and fruit impart bio-energetic elements to us that help sustain our subtle life forces and renew the spirit. Cooked grains are dead food. Processed sugars are perverted food.

Only Nature's raw vegetables and fruits are the optimal, universal carbohydrate food for human nutrition.

Here we are beginning to discover that, if our diet is too rich in cooked grains and processed foods, then our health will be less than if raw vegetables and fruit were included. This does not mean that we do not use cooked grains. Grains offer superior nutrition compared to many other diets we could discuss, such as the martini and barbecue diet. Everything is relative. When we want the best of the best in every meal, raw and lightly steamed vegetables will be on the plate. By applying the 12 Optimal Nutrition Factors, we can quickly set the standard for our health.

Right now, this information can empower you to improve your nutrition.

- If you are a grain eater, add some salad.
- Snack on some fruit.
- If you are a meat and potato person, add some salad.
- If you don't eat vegetables, start now!

How Much Carbohydrate Do I Need Every Day?

Carbohydrate is not stored in any significant quantity in the body. A tiny bit is stored as glycogen, a concentrated from of glucose for times of emergency when access to a burst of energy is needed for survival. Even though carbohydrates are not stored in the body, and since carbohydrates are the most abundant component of many people's diets, obtaining them for energy is not a critical concern. It is highly unlikely to find a person with a nutritional deficiency of carbohydrates, whereas we do find people deficient in the other macro-nutrients such as protein, essential fatty acids (oils), as well as micronutrients – vitamins and minerals.

Currently, there is no Required Daily Allowance for carbohydrates because it is so abundant and the body has so many ways to make it. For fat-weight loss purposes, it makes sense to set the minimum standard at whatever level it takes to avoid muscle loss and excessive ketosis – the processing of stored fat to meet the glucose needs of the body. Excessive ketosis causes the loss of sodium, a critical cation (a positive-charged ion) of cellular nutrition, and interferes with the core of cellular function. Dehydration also occurs. Often, to initiate a fat-burning metabolism, carbohydrate intake is restricted to 30 grams per day, temporarily. With adequate carbohydrate, which often is as little as 45-60 grams a day, ketosis can be controlled or modified to burn fat without causing muscle loss and without sending the body into the altered metabolism of survival. This would set the extreme low but safe marker for carbohydrate intake.

But what is the *optimal* level of carbohydrate intake for the daily diet? It might be 120-180 grams per day (athletes will need more), depending on serveral factors:

- glucose metabolism
- ratio of macro-nutrients
- activity level
- body weight
- age
- gender
- digestion

These factors also must be taken into account during a weight reduction program.

Some researchers claim that 80% of a person's total dietary calories should come from carbohydrates. This is common with a vegetarian regimen. There is a simple way to figure the optimal level of dietary carbohydrate intake. Just calculate the body's protein requirement, then correlate that to glucose metabolism, which can be qualified and quantified via the FitTest. The result is a ratio of carbohydrate to protein to fat that serves the body with a balanced metabolism and sustained energy.

The misnamed "healthy heart" diet plans promote a high carbohydrate, low protein, low fat diet that often is 75% carbohydrate, 20% protein, and 5% fat. Other researchers promote a 40% ratio of carbohydrates and then advocate that 30% should come from protein and 30% from fat. Although this popular 40-30-30 plan is an improvement to the appalling statistics of the *high* carbohydrate plans, even the very best one-size-fits-all dietary plans are only working for a third of the people that do them.

So what is the key to better odds of success? Of course, it's **individualization**. Even more than individualizing the amounts of foods according to muscle mass or body weight and then fitting it in to a one-size-fits-all ratio, *individualization according to the metabolic sensitivity to carbohydrates can tailor your program for greater accuracy.* You could be a 35-35-30 person, or even a 30-30-40 person, or a 35-40-25 person. And, yes, there are some "lucky dogs" that can thrive on a 50-30-20 diet of carbohydrate-to-protein-to-fat ratios.

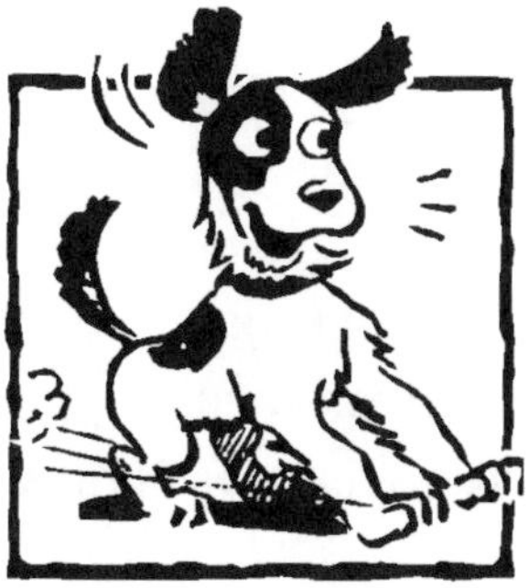

Thus, a lab test, such as the FitTest can help fine-tune your diet for the most optimal weight and health. Then, by applying the nutritional insights presented here, you can enjoy the best foods and the best nutrition and literally re-sculpt your body and revitalize your health.

How Do Carbohydrates Contribute to Dietary Fiber?

Fiber is an underrated component of food. It naturally occurs in substantial quantities in vegetables, grains, beans and fruit. Fiber helps the body control the uptake of sugar and fats. It buffers proteins to protect the body from their acidic qualities. It helps with the removal of toxins from the bowel, and provides the correct terrain for the pro-biotic organisms that inhabit the bowel such as acidophilus, bifidus, and bulgaricus. In addition, it helps bulk the stool and balance the water content for proper elimination function.

The cornerstone of many of the successful, natural cholesterol-reducing programs is a fiber supplement. It only makes sense because fiber controls a portion of the insulin response as well as intake of fat. The reason people need a fiber supplement is that the refining of carbohydrate foods (to make cereals, flour, sugar, and white rice) removes the fiber, creating a deficiency of the much-needed fiber.

Why Are Vegetables Essential for a Healthy Life?

Stop and think for a moment. When you prepare a meal, do you first plan its meat or starch portion? Is it like, "Let's see, I have a lamb roast. What do I have to go with it?" Or do you proceed in this way, "Let's have spaghetti. I hope I have some garlic bread and olives to go with it." If these are your natural thought processes, then your food plan is *not* prioritized to focus on optimal health.

On the other hand, if your focus on food is, "I have beautiful fresh salad. I think that some spaghetti on the side would be fun." Or, "Look at this fine organic broccoli. I think I'll make a sesame-miso sauce and have it with a bit of fish." With these approaches your orientation is geared towards vegetables and health.

Vegetables, mostly raw, some cooked, are the essential element for health through nutrition when combined with an optimal balance of protein and fat.

"What's for dinner, Mom?"

"Broccoli, salad and broiled trout, dear."

Many people say that they don't particularly like vegetables. They, instead, prefer smoked meats, spicy sauces, tangy cheeses or sweet desserts over the common and ordinary vegetable. It is un-

Health Tip: When preparing a meal, pick your vegetables first. Make meat, fats, and starches a side dish.

derstandable that vegetables can taste bland and boring to sophisticated people whose taste buds have been titillated by salt, spices, chemical flavors, sugar and smoke. Like an addiction, constant overstimulation of the taste buds with strong impulses – particularly chemical tastes – can alter the sense of taste and establish a need for strong taste sensations. For instance, some people can become mildly addicted to hot peppers as the pain of eating them causes the release of endorphins in the brain and thus imparts a feeling of well being. *Viva el jalapeño!* Beyond that, the onslaught of sugar and hidden sugar, as well as tobacco and coffee, dull the sense of taste.

Sadly, most people today have lost the ability to enjoy a bite of crisp carrot, sweet juicy corn, earthy sprouts and chewy cabbage. Some people have even lost the desire and ability to enjoy fresh fruits, and thus miss the sour, but luscious, sensation of biting into a ripe plum or the aromatic explosion of chomping down on a crisp apple. When the natural ability to taste fresh and subtle flavors becomes jaded, or warped, due to the onslaught of "dead" foods doctored with additives to make them palatable, people find the basic, wholesome foods less palatable. Please do not interpret this as a hint for a bland diet. Peppers, herbs and spices enhance foods tastefully and nutritionally. Here in Texas we say, "A day without salsa is like a day without salsa!" Not exactly the most profound observation, but food is meant to be tasted and enjoyed.

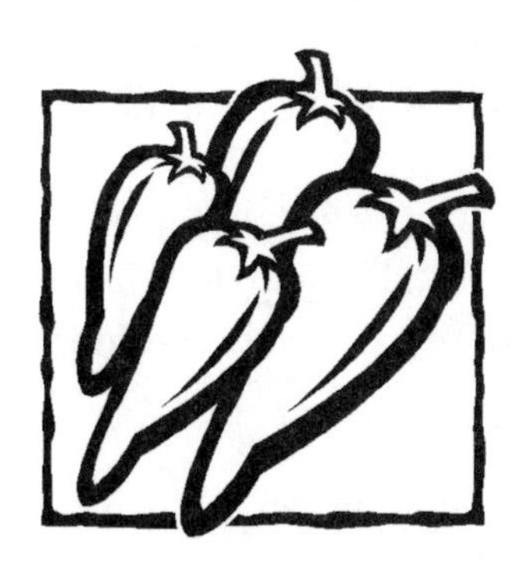

In the natural health field, it is common knowledge that the flavors of fresh, organically grown vegetables are exquisite for a person in a healthy state. Imagine the wonderful, fresh crunch of sweet celery; the tang and flavor explosion of a slice of red bell pepper; the touch of tart lemon juice; the sweet, smooth taste of jicama; the pungent essence of fresh basil; the surprising bite of a piece of radish; the prickly aroma of parsley; and the crisp coolness of green leafy lettuce. All of these vegetables impart their precious waters, enzymes, vitamins and minerals to help our body's cells thrive!

Several factors in commercial farming and current food preparation methods explain why we are not able to enjoy the subtle flavors of many vegetables and fruits.

- Commercial farming and synthetic fertilizers have given us an object that merely looks like a carrot or a peach. It may be jumbo in size, flawless of skin, but it is hollow in nutrients. The commercial vegetables and fruit do not contain their full flavor, due to the absence of important trace minerals and the plant's full, natural vitality. Further, "vine-ripened" produce possesses the most astounding tastes as opposed to the picked-green, force-ripened with chemicals, or never-ripened-fully produce that fills the bins at the grocery store.
- Because commercially grown foods often taste and look less than appetizing, the food industry adds synthetic colors and waxes to trick our eyes.
- When the food is prepared, many people add sugar and spices to provide the taste sensation we inherently know the food should have.
- Processed foods contain chemicals and additives which can overstimulate our sense of taste.
- Hybridized foods are grown to increase the sugar content so the taste buds are stimulated with extra sweet.

I have an unequivocal guarantee for you, if you are a person who currently shuns vegetables. As you reintroduce a variety of fresh vegetables into your diet and decrease the chemical overstimulation of your taste buds, the vegetables will taste better and better every day. In their natural state, organic foods are vibrant with delicious and subtle flavors that make the body naturally desire them. Nutrition should be exciting, flavorful and satisfying to all of our senses: sight, smell, taste, feel and even sound (crunch!).

The good news is that the lost taste faculty will readily return when we follow a more natural food plan. If we can just get through the transition period, as a person must with any addictive process before coming clean, we will receive the reward of rediscovering wonderful "new" taste sensations that are completely fulfilling.

How extreme do you have to be? Some people worry that I'm trying to turn them into a rabbit. Not so. Remember to keep everything in a balanced perspective. The simple belabored message here is to add vegetables to each meal. Learn to appreciate a variety of vegetables. Keep it simple.

Case History – Diabetes Reversal With Diet, Nutritional Therapy

The power of this dietary plan is awesome. It is the first step a person experiencing adult-onset diabetes should take. Here is a case history.

Subject: Male, age 48, height - 6', weight - 240 lbs. (overweight) Father was diabetic. Maternal grandmother was diabetic.

Symptoms: Fasting blood glucose 245 mg/dl.

After being diagnosed as Diabetic, Type II, he had a 30-day grace period to control it dietarily, before being given oral medication. He was told this was strictly a genetic disease and that he would inevitably need medication.

In **March, '98** began the *Pro-Vita!* Plan along with a custom-designed multi-vitamin, multi-mineral supplement (Custom Essentials), as well as nutritional (herbal) support for the pancreas and liver.

Six weeks later, in **April, '98,** he reported:

- Felt better within 3 days
- Lost six pounds (was not eating any refined sugar, deleted coffee)
- Blood glucose 115 mg/dl (still higher than is safe, but a major improvement)
- Incidences of night-sweats diminished

The program continued unabated and, in **May '98**, he reported:

- Lost six more pounds
- Reflexes faster
- Blood glucose 102 mg/dl (within normal range)
- Energy much better. More energy in evening. Bowling regularly.

In **June, '98**, the herbal supplements were stopped. By **November '98**, weight was stable for his large frame at a fit 188 lbs. All monthly tests of glucose were in the normal range.

What happened to the genetic, inevitable decline into adult onset diabetes? Evidently, diet was predisposing him to diabetes. When the diet was changed, his body was able to adapt and return to a normal carbohydrate metabolism. The natural therapies accelerated the improvement and increased his adaptability and metabolic self-regulation. The herbal supplements provided specific nutritional factors for key organ systems. Thus, the program was comprehensive, and the body responded quickly with a more optimal state of health.

This is not a unique occurrence. Every nutritionist I know has cases of helping people with carbohydrate metabolism problems. Overshadowing this discussion, I can still hear Dr. Wheelwright shouting from the podium, *"You are not a doughboy! Your body is protein, fat and minerals with less than 6% carbohydrate in transit for energy! Why would you want to base your diet on carbohydrates, and neglect the very nutrients you're made out of?"* Food for thought!

CHAPTER THIRTEEN

Carbohydrates: Health and Fat Loss Tips

The Big Appetite and the Sweet Tooth

When beginning a new program, the body often tries to stay in its established comfort zone. The body sometimes resists changes – even changes that **shift** health **right** in the positive direction. If a person has an appetite that is accustomed to refined sugars, that person's metabolic processes are geared to that fuel. When such a person has a perfect meal that establishes a balanced, but different, hormonal response, the body recognizes it as different. This difference means a period of adaptation and change. This new diet does not jam in the insulin response. The hunger center in the brain that I previously referred to as the "sweet tooth" is accustomed to being satisfied by massive amounts of sugar. Now, with a proper diet, that sugar is not there. The body has to digest or "work" a little to derive its glucose.

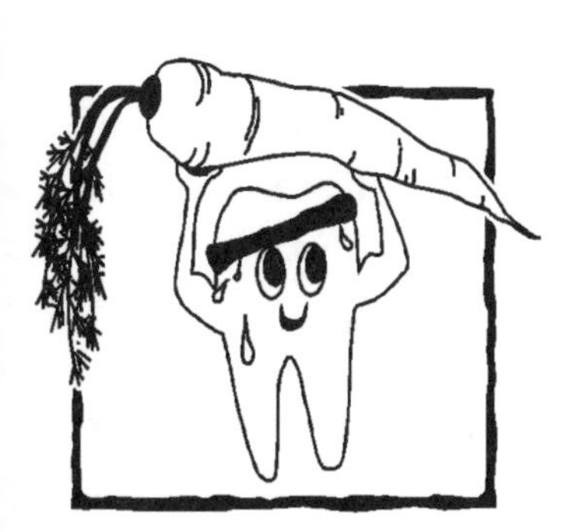

The brain can turn on a request for jelly beans rather than re-tool the body's metabolism to burn a slower-access, more complex fuel. This is simply the acting-out of an acquired bad habit. **A person can have a big appetite and be temporarily hungry even though all nutritional factors have been perfectly met. At this point, it is best to have a plan.**

When I personally experienced this phenomenon, I asked Dr. Stuart Wheelwright what to do. *He had me eat lightly steamed kale with breakfast.* Why that worked, I do not know. But I've seen it work for many other people. Perhaps that's a little strange for you, so fear not, I have an additional plan. Dr. Wheelwright explained to me that, in his opinion, the brain had a center that responded to the three macro-nutrients via certain hormones. This center's most dominant receptor site would respond to carbohydrates, but there was another site for fat. *He felt that if beneficial fats were included in a meal, the brain would have the feeling of fullness and be satisfied.* He speculated that there was a center for protein as well, but that it was easily overridden by the sugar center.

Seven years after Dr. Wheelwright's death, science discovered the hormone, *leptin* that tells the appetite to "calm down, there is enough nutrition for the body to function properly". Also, there is an intestinal hormone, Cholecystokinin (CCK), that curbs the appetite, especially when fats are eaten. It seems to interact with seratonin to regulate hunger. *Thus, fats in the diet* are *what turn off the appetite*. The body is programmed to feel full and satisfied when fats are in the meal. Prior to the Industrial Revolution, fats were natural-source lipids from plants and animals. Now, fats are often highly processed, altered molecules such as partially-hydrogenated oils. They still satisfy the appetite, but bring health problems as we have discussed.

When you begin harnessing your body's fat burning mechanism via a properly balanced diet, it is easy to resist the "I feel hungry even though I just ate the most nutritious meal of my life" syndrome. Here are a couple of simple solutions.

- Have a balanced food bar (compatible with your lab results) with a piece of celery, salad, jicama, or other raw vegetable.

- Tough it out with will power. The "Gee, I'd love a cookie syndrome" only lasts a few days for most people, anyway. After that, you are "Free! Free! Free!" of the inner pang for a food that unravels your health as proper hormonal balance reclaims the metabolism.
- For the few people who have a strong "genetic" desire for sweets meaning that they are susceptible to sweet cravings which is often accompanied by emotional needs for sweets, the best advice is to allow yourself fruit. Use fresh, raw fruits that are low on the glycemic index such as apples, pears, peaches, plums, grapefruit, oranges, nectarines, grapes, cherries, kiwi, blackberries, blueberries, and strawberries. Avoid high glycemic fruits such as raisins, dates, banana, papaya and mango. This transitional strategy will prevent the "all-or-nothing" approach that is actually a fight against yourself.

This table includes foods which gallop into the bloodstream so fast that they often startle the pancreas.

Sugar "Whoas"

Avoid these foods to help harness your fat-burning metabolism. (See the substitution information in Chapter 20.) Just Say "Whoa!" to:

Refined Sugar	Granulated sugar, Sugared drinks, Cookies, Pastries, Candy, Desserts, Canned foods listing "sugar" in the ingredients
Refined flour products	White bread, Pasta, Dumplings, Crackers
Refined starches	Instant potatoes, Rice cakes, Corn flakes, Potato chips, Corn chips, Cereals, Microwave-baked potatoes and Minute rice

Three Misconceptions About Carbohydrates

The following text dispels three common types of misinformation about carbohydrates. The three misconceptions here do not mean that carbohydrates are a bad food. They do not mean that carbohydrates are to blame. The misconceptions are included here so you can see through the dietary myths and build a dietary foundation for optimal health. It's not the carbohydrates, it's the imbalance between carbohydrates, protein, and fat that contributes to poor energy (stamina), heart disease, and obesity. With *The Weight Is Over* program, you'll receive the optimal ratios of macro-nutrients for your individual metabolism, so you can balance carbohydrates with protein and fats and avoid these problems.

Misconception #1: Carbohydrates are the food for athletes.

One misconception about carbohydrates is that the muscles burn glucose (a carbohydrate) for energy. This misconception has lead athletes to "carb-loading" practices where they load up on carbohydrates before a big event by eating pasta, bread, and rice. It has also lead to the image that when athletes work out and are thirsty, they need to slam down a Gator Aid©, Coke©, or Pepsi© as good nutrition for their energy needs.

Why is this a misconception? Because *muscles burn fat, along with a little glucose.* It is the fat that gives the muscles stamina and endurance, as well as helps the quick energy fuel, glucose, last longer. *Drinking high sugar beverages locks out the muscles' access to fat and forces them to run on the superficial, high-octane glucose.*

A gram of carbohydrates yields four calories of cellular fuel, making carbohydrates an easily accessible, quick energy fuel source as compared to the slower access of protein and fat. It works for a while, but soon the glucose must be replenished. Every time the sugar drink is used, the pancreas must secrete insulin to make the glucose available to the cells. Thus, "carb-loading" and use of sugared drinks wears out the pancreas and causes insulin-related problems such as diabetes, hypoglycemia, obesity, hypertension, and elevated cholesterol.

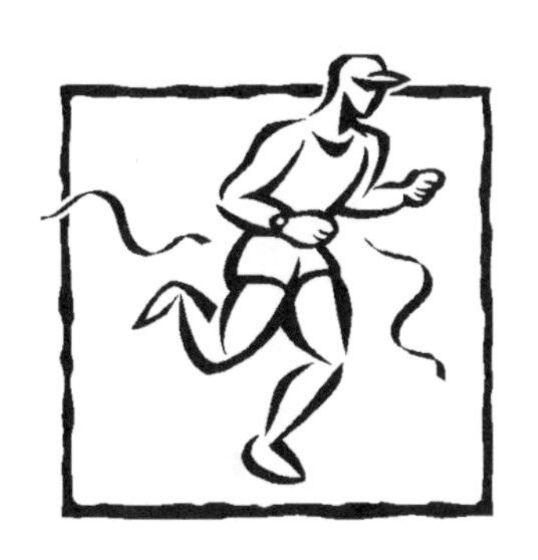

Here is an example. In 1993, an Australian marathon runner came to me for nutritional counsel for peak performance. He said, "God gave me a special talent – running. I love to run. I do it well. I don't understand why I can't improve my time. My knees are strong. I set records in the first 12 to 15 miles. But I lose it toward the end. My final sprint is pathetic." [I could hear the Vangelis music from the movie "Chariots of Fire."] He certainly was passionate about running; in fact, he was on fire to win the Austin Marathon coming in three months.

I replied that it might just be an issue of stamina based on biochemistry and bio-energy. To this regard, I counseled that he try the *Pro-Vita!* meals, lay off the excessive sugar drinks, and quit making carbohydrates the foundation of his diet so there would be a better balance in his diet.

He noticed results within two weeks. Greater stamina and endurance in the latter miles, especially miles 20 to 26, allowed for a consistently improving time. He still had the ability to sprint at the end, based on better conservation of glucose, because the diet now provided a better balance of protein and fat. Over the next two months, he made consistent improvement in running. There is more to this story regarding his performance in the marathon, but I'll continue it soon in a later chapter.

Misconception #2: Carbohydrate-based diets are good for the heart.

Another misconception about carbohydrates is that they are good for the heart. This myth has been taught to us under the guise of the "healthy heart" diet of low fat, low protein, high carbohydrate. The glaring statistics of increased heart and cardiovascular disease, even in people who exercise and eat pasta, is enough to make us reconsider making carbohydrates the foundation of a diet plan.

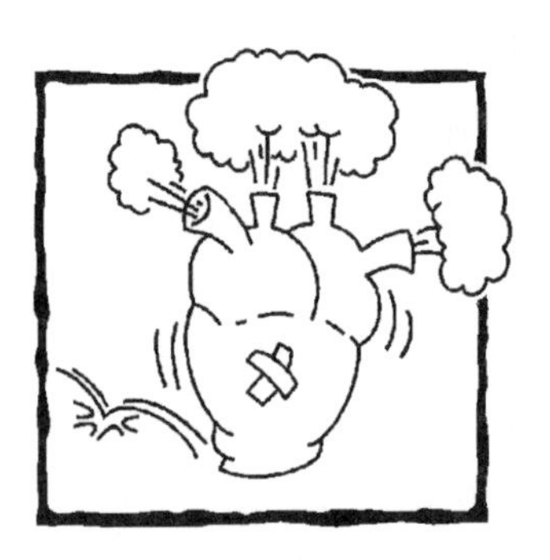

In the 1980's, the dietary push toward high complex carbohydrate (grain) intake began. The trends showing that this is not the dietary answer are quite evident, as America has increased in obesity and heart disease on a high carbohydrate diet. A carbohydrate food plan does not build the quality tissues required for optimal health. Also, carbohydrates such as grains often become allergenic if used excessively. This may be caused by modern hybridization and agricultural methods rather than the natural grain. Carbohydrates are a survival food and will do if no other food is available. Yet, most people want more than "make-do" with foods since foods have the potential to build a more optimal level of health. Ultimately, high complex carbohydrate diets do not suffice for good health, particularly if vegetables are neglected.

A man consulted with me for heart-related concerns. He had a heart attack two years prior, and now was found to have 90% blockage of the coronary arteries. His diet for the past two years had been "healthy heart" based on grains and pasta with sincere avoidance of meat, fat, and alcohol. He was not expected to live long. Here's what he has to say,

I am 58 years old and I feel fortunate to be here. Seven years ago I had a heart attack and received five by-passes. For years I have been into natural health and thought I knew a little about diet. I was always very athletic so I thought high carb was the way to go. Well, I was wrong. In just three very short years after the by-passes, on that diet I was plugged up in two more arteries, 70 and 80%, and high sugar [elevated glucose 300]. I got on Dr. Tips' Pro-Vita! Plan and in three months I was so improved that I was able to travel abroad to the Holy Land – a lifetime dream. The medical opinion promoting the high carb diet could not be further from the truth. We thank you for our lives. – Edward Lake, TN

Misconception #3: Cut back on fat and protein (because it contains fat), and increase carbohydrate to lose weight.

A third area where carbohydrates are misunderstood is regarding weight loss. Many people think that if they cut back on fat, cut back on protein because it is often associated with fat, and eat grains and pasta, which are low in fat, that they will lose the fat around their waists. But this carbohydrate-based diet has not proven to do this. In fact, over the past 12 years that America has been shunning fat and eating more carbohydrates, the country has gained 10 pounds per adult person!

One day, a lady came to the clinic for counsel. She had been a vegetarian for many years and presented the following symptoms: obesity, low self-esteem, low energy, poor muscle tone, weak digestion, and abdominal bloating. I asked her, "Tell me about your diet." and she replied, "I eat bread, grains, rice, potatoes, fruit, millet, cereals, salads. I have a very, very healthy diet. I keep fats to a minimum, but I can't lose weight. I don't even eat large quantities."

She was misinformed about carbohydrates and this misinformation was costing her a great deal. Neither she nor I could determine where the myths that she should avoid fat and protein originated, but she was well on her way to chronic degenerative disease while eating whole, healthy, vegetarian foods. By adding other healthy vegetarian foods – germinated seeds, miso, cottage cheese, feta cheese, olive oil, grapeseed oil, and avocado – to her diet, she increased the protein and fat. By reducing starch and capitalizing on vegetables, she reduced the excessive carbohydrates. She first began regaining her tissue integrity and muscle tone. Then she began losing weight. Then her energy improved and she became an avid rowing enthusiast.

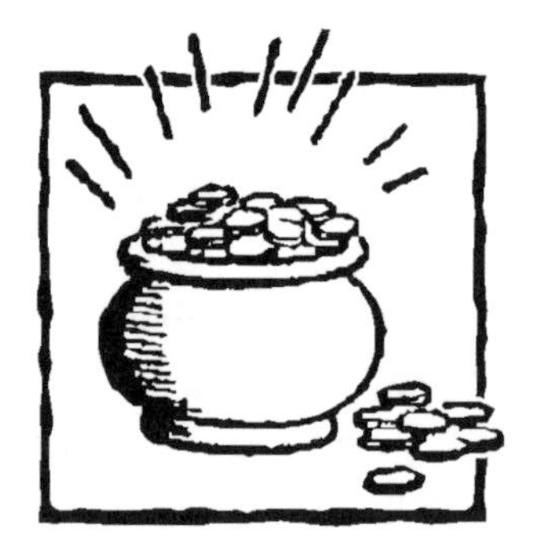

Whew! There you have it – refined golden nuggets of information about macro-nutrients. We're ready to move on to Part Three, which presents key insights on factors other than macro-nutrients that bring success in fat-reduction and in improving health. It will help you tailor your diet to your specific goals.

Part Three

Tips To Help You Go The Distance And Win

CHAPTER FOURTEEN

Self Tests – Is Your Digestion Healthy?

All diseases start on your plate.
– Old Naturopathic Aphorism

We must take a moment here to discuss the very foundation of natural health – *digestion*, and its flip side – *elimination*. Volumes have been written about the critical importance of digestion, because it is the body's beginning of nutrition. More than the fact that digestion (the breaking down of food molecules for absorption into our bodies) is at the heart of health and disease, we must have good digestion to lose fat-weight effectively. Volumes have also been written about the critical importance of elimination because of the poor health that results when there is poor waste removal. One such volume is *Your Liver – Your Lifeline*, (Tips, 1986) a book that brings new insights to this age old issue, but for the sake of brevity, we'll leave the nutritional and naturopathic information between its covers. More than the fact that elimination (the removal of wastes) is essential for good health, we cannot lose fat-weight effectively without that system's cooperation. Therefore, both digestion and elimination are critically important to fat-weight loss.

Effective digestion and elimination are critical factors in fat-weight reduction.

We are faced with the simple premise that in order to have a proper macro-nutrient balance, we must have effective digestion of protein, carbohydrates, and fats. We don't have to be rocket scientists to understand that basic fact, so this premise is somewhat obvious. Thus, with all the talk about grams of food and calories of energy, we're really confronted with this simple fact: It's not how many grams of protein, fat, and carbohydrate we eat; *it's how many molecules we digest, assimilate and humanize for use at the cellular level that sets the standard of our health and impacts our fat-burning mechanism.*

With that understanding, the big issue is this. Over 70% of the American population have some kind of gastro-intestinal disorder. Antacids sell several billion dollars of product annually, and, according to many nutritionists, they contribute to a worsening of the overall digestive processes. Poor digestion is pandemic among people who eat an unnatural diet.

If you have digestive problems, now is the time to help your body correct this problem because it is the termites in your foundation, the worm-rot in your hull, the rust in your chassis. It is quietly undermining your health. The information in this book will help you eat so your digestion can be restored. Proper eating will correct a majority of the digestive concerns in this country. [Note to self: if 10 million people read *The Weight Is Over* or *The Pro-Vita! Plan for Optimal Nutrition* or *Eating Energy,* sell stock in antacid companies.]

To assist you in quantifying your digestive system, here are two questionnaires to help you focus on digestive function. The first questionnaire focuses on a hyper or over-functioning of the digestive processes. The second questionnaire focuses on a hypo or under-functioning digestive system.

Hyperactive Digestion

Is your digestive system overproducing?

Overactive Digestive System Questionnaire	Y or N
1. Ulcers, or history of ulcers?	___
2. Dark or black stool (if not on supplemental iron)	___
3. Belching relieves bloating, indigestion	___
4. Drinking milk relieves heartburn	___
5. History of gastritis (stomach inflammation)	___
6. Craves carbonated beverages that bring relief	___
7. Frequently has heartburn	___
8. Must use antacids frequently	___
9. Feels emotions in stomach	___
10. Indigestion often interrupts sleep	___
11. Nervous feeling in stomach	___
12. Loud gurgling in stomach	___
13. Stomach pains	___
14, Stomach ache when thinking of food, before meals	___
15. Smoker	___
16. Frequent abdominal pains	___
17. Acid indigestion	___
18. Reflux	___
19. Regurgitation of food, esophagus spasms	___
20. Heat or burning in stomach	___

If you answered 4 or more Yes, there is a likelihood that you experience a hyper or overactive digestion.

Hypoactive Digestion

Next is a questionnaire to help determine if your digestion is underactive. This can result in poor digestion and absorption of nutrients as well as imbalances in the intestinal flora. Is your digestive system under-producing?

Underactive Digestive System Questionnaire	Y or N
1. Burping after meals	___
2. Bloating after meals	___
3. Allergic reactions to food (fatigue, sinus congestion)	___
4. Diagnosed food allergies	___
5. Too full after eating a moderate amount	___
6. Constipation	___
7. Use laxatives frequently	___
8. Appetite, low	___
9. Queasy stomach occurs frequently	___
10. Stomach "knots" when eating nuts	___
11. Frequent gas (flatulence)	___
12. Hard stools, straining	___

If you answered 3 or more Yes, you may have a weak digestion and are not effectively processing foods into useable nutrients.

Natural treatments for digestive concerns are very effective. Most people respond well to the addition of digestive enzyme products along with a pro-biotic supplement of acidophilus, bifidus, and bulgaricus (the beneficial microorganisms that inhabit the intestines). Others require laboratory testing for pancreatic enzyme deficiencies, dysbiosis (harmful microorganisms in the intestines) and parasites.

Elimination System Function

Regarding bowel elimination, constipation and/or frequent diarrhea is also pandemic in cultures that base their diets on refined, processed, and denatured foods. Faulty elimination results in a buildup of toxicity at the cellular level. Like New Yorker's during the garbage strike, the body is not happy when the wastes are not removed. Cellular toxicity is a basis for aging, free-radical pathologies (cancer) and bacterial and viral infections.

Here is a questionnaire to help you focus on any need to improve your eliminative processes. Is your elimination system working properly?

Elimination System Function Questionnaire	Y or N
1. Constipation	___
2. Diarrhea, chronic	___
3. Alternating constipation/diarrhea	___
4. Fiber supplements cause constipation	___
5. Mucous in stools	___
6. Lower abdominal cramps	___
7. Spastic colon	___
8. Irritable bowel disorder	___
9. Poorly formed stool	___
10. Acne, pimples, skin eruptions	___
11. Vaginal yeast overgrowth	___
12. Recurrent infections	___
13. More than three stools a day	___
14. Indigestion occurs 2 hours after eating	___
15. Seasonal diarrhea	___

16. Food allergies ___
17. Foul-smelling stool ___
18. Dry skin and hair ___
19. Gas, flatulence ___
20. Fatigue after meals ___
21. Sheen on stool ___
22. Trouble gaining weight ___
23. History of antibiotic use ___

If you answered 4 or more Yes, improvements in bowel function and intestinal tissue integrity can provide advantages to your health.

Many nutritionists recommend intestinal supplements such as fiber, cleansing formulas, and pro-biotic formulas to improve bowel function and intestinal tissue integrity. Some people carry several pounds of old fecal matter in their colons. Cleansing the colon can play a major role in fat-weight loss as well as overall health.

While preparing to lose weight via your FitTest results, it can be very beneficial to add a digestive supplement and a colon cleansing supplement to prepare your body for proper digestion, assimilation of nutrients, and elimination of waste materials with simple supplementation.

CHAPTER FIFTEEN

Water's Role in Fat Loss and Health

The natural healing force within us is the greatest force in getting well.
– Hippocrates

Water: The Elixir Vitae (The Tonic of Life)

Drinking pure water is a healing and rejuvenating therapy, particularly for people who chronically do not drink enough. Proper water intake provides numerous benefits and even cures very serious problems.

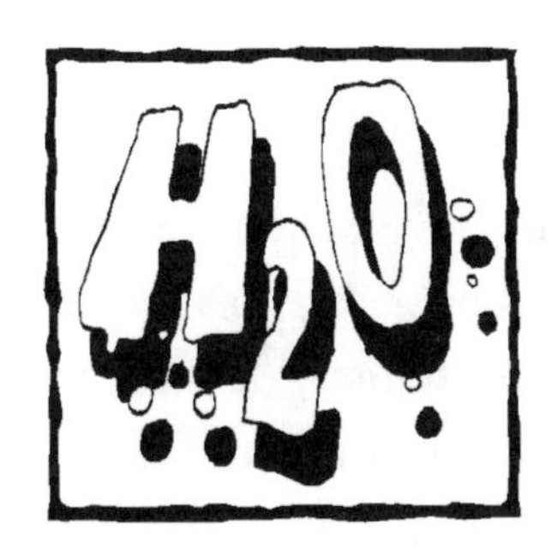

The astounding simplicity is that pure water is one of your premier fat-loss potions!

The key to fat loss is first, being able to burn fat, and second, being able to dispose of the metabolic by-products. If you are even a little bit dehydrated, your body will not effectively burn fat. Water is a necessary ingredient in the reduction of fat because it helps eliminate ketones, a by-product of fat combustion. Since ketones can be used in lieu of glucose for energy, the faster you eliminate them, the faster you lose weight.

Water, Huh? Plain and Simple.

It may seem too simple to cite the virtues of water, but frankly, much of the information in this entire book is presented because of our deviations from the basic principles of health, also called Natural Law. We must look at the water issue as yet another area where the apple cart of health has tipped over and we're losing the fundamental basis of our lives. Again, if this material can inspire you to ShiftRight into better water drinking habits, that change will pay you a huge dividend in your overall health as well as help you lose fat-weight.

Why? Well let's begin with the fact that your body is 75% water, making water by far the main component of your body. Now, for fun, think of your favorite Hollywood screen idol. That person is mostly a bag of water with lard on top (their brain). What about you and me? Oh, well. So much for an exaggerated self-opinion.

Now, what is the quality of the water that is the cradle of our metabolic activities, tissues, and blood? Is it polluted with chemicals from tap water? Is it coffee, sodas, artificially-flavored drinks? Or is it the vital, nascent water in fruit and vegetables? Is it clean, sparkling water from the Earth?

Water is the universal solvent. In the body, it picks up toxins and the metabolic by-products of fat combustion and takes them to the kidneys for excretion. Thus, water is our primary detoxification agent at the cellular level. If we do not have enough water, the kidneys cannot perform their job. The body recognizes when it is short of water and will retain water, causing the kidneys to detoxify fewer pollutants from the blood.

Low water intake puts the brakes on fat metabolism. When the kidneys do not detoxify the blood properly because of low water intake, the detoxification burden falls back to the liver. To accomplish fat-loss, we depend on our livers to metabolize stored fat. If the liver is occupied with pollutants that the kidneys could have handled, it metabolizes less fat. The obvious priority is to protect the body from potentially life-threatening toxins.

With a good flow of pure water through your body, you can lose more weight. Your ability to metabolize fat floats on the rocking waves of water. The more metabolic by-products (ketones) you eliminate, the faster your body can access more stored fat to burn.

The solution to pollution is dilution.

In a toxic environment, the body stores water in its extracellular matrix (the space between the cells) to dilute the poisons. What does the body need to detoxify itself? Water. The foremost answer to simple water retention is to drink more water! When the body's environment is detoxified, it will no longer store water in its matrix. This simple paradox can spare many people the trap of taking a diuretic and forcing water (along with precious potassium) out of the body, only to have the body replace the lost water as soon as it can. When the body has a constant supply of pure water for detoxification, it will release stored water when it perceives it is safe.

What Is The Right Amount of Water?

The right amount of water varies from person to person. It depends on body weight, activity level, perspiration, water content of foods, temperature, and a host of other factors. Overweight people need more water than thin ones. Thus, the platitude, "Drink 8 glasses of water a day," is merely a ballpark concept. It steers us in the right direction.

During the time you are dedicated to fat loss and *The Weight Is Over* program, you can determine your water intake by your water outflow. Here is your rule: drink enough water to urinate between nine and twelve times a day. Drink until you slosh! It's best to drink water over the course of the day, not in giant gulps. For fat-burning, if you are not urinating three times every four waking hours, you need to increase your water intake, or you will not be burning as much fat as you potentially could be.

Water! There is no substitute. Not coffee, not sodas, not tea, not bottled fruit juice. The body has a need for pure water, pure and simple.

The best way to achieve this volume of water is to get a sports bottle and drink it dry frequently. Make a goal to empty the bottle by a certain time in the morning. Refill it and do it again. There is a saying about water and weight loss – "*When you feel thirsty, it's already too late!*" This means is that when your body gets around to triggering a thirst signal, you are already dehydrated and your fat-burning mechanism has already been inhibited. This is why a commitment to drinking water frequently and routinely is important during a fat-loss program.

What Is The Right Water To Drink?

Rather than go into a detailed discussion of tap vs. distilled vs. spring vs. bottled waters, let's have one simple rule. Avoid tap water. It's unfit to drink. Most tap water contains over 200 trace chemicals, ranging from industrial pollutants and agricultural poisons to chemical additives such as chlorine and fluoride. These trace chemicals are linked with allergies and inhibited immune systems. Some of the other trace toxins in water can react with chlorine to form carcinogenic compounds. Further, chlorine and fluoride inhibit the action of Vitamin E and increase the likelihood of free-radical oxidation, a process that contributes to aging and chronic-degenerative diseases.

Without belaboring this point, detoxification is an important part of proper weight loss. So don't keep adding toxins. Be

Rule of Thumb: Don't drink tap water unless there is no other water to drink.

thankful that municipal water systems helped eliminate plagues and infectious diseases by killing water-borne microorganisms. But don't drink tap water. Instead, use bottled, reverse-osmosis, alkaline water, or even distilled water. Drink pure water so it can perform as the universal solvent and flush unwanted or toxic molecules from your body.

Health and Fat Loss Tips

Several people I have consulted with used this method to increase their pure water intake. They bought cases of reputable bottled water in small bottles of 11 or 12 ounces each. Then they simply drank one for every waking hour. One man set the alarm on his wristwatch to beep hourly to remind him to slam down a small bottle of water. The results were amazing. Also, these dedicated water imbibers did not experience the headaches, bad breath, and fatigue some people experience when losing weight.

Water is a powerful tool for health and especially for fat-burning weight loss. Put it to work for you right now. Again, do this one step now. **Line 'em up, drink 'em down.** Drinking water throughout the day will start you on your pathway to an increased fat-burning metabolism and better health.

CHAPTER SIXTEEN

Exercise's Role in Fat Loss and Health

To maintain good health, the body must be exercised properly (stretching, brisk walking, biking, swimming, deep breathing, good posture, etc.) and nourished wisely (natural foods), to maintain a normal weight and increase the good life of radiant health, joy and happiness.
– Paul Bragg

Although this is primarily a nutrition book, the importance of exercise cannot be ignored. In fact, in many ways, diet and exercise are inseparable, as we will discuss. In a primitive society, exercise probably was not a problem. People just got their daily exercise naturally, mainly in their daily work. Our sedentary lifestyles with automobiles, elevators and desk jobs make some sort of exercise routine vital for health. Let's look briefly at how *The Weight Is Over* can increase the benefits of exercise and vice versa.

What are the benefits of exercise?

- Muscles are made to be exercised. In this way they receive new nutrients and discard waste products.
- Exercise is essential to move proteins out of the lymphatic system into the cells where they can rebuild and renew life at the cellular level.
- The temporary increase in body temperature caused by exercise kills (pasteurizes) viruses and bacteria, making exercise an important immune system support.

- Muscles burn fat and exercise makes the muscles burn more fat. Resistance exercise builds more muscle to burn more fat.

As an attitude adjustment, we should not separate exercise and diet. Without a proper diet, exercise will not bring the benefits we expect. It will not provide the key to fat-loss. In fact, it may simply cause more stress as the effects of oxidation increase during exercise. On the other hand, a proper diet without exercise will not bring the optimal effect either. The two need to work together.

The Case For Mild Exercise Such As Walking

If you are a person who hates exercise and would like to exorcise exercise, do not despair. The latest research on exercise and health shows that going for a walk can accomplish most of what strenuous running, boring workouts, and other forms of "no pain, no gain" programs aim to achieve. Thus, a simple daily walk provides tremendous health, fat-loss, and cardiovascular benefits. It raises your basal metabolism to burn fat more effectively as well as circulate the nutrients that build muscle and detoxify wastes. It is the basic form of exercise, the minimal, but effective, commitment you should make to yourself.

Of course, you will not build marathon stamina or sculpt a Schwarzenegger physique by walking. There are still benefits of more strenuous programs for those who earn them. But for our purposes regarding weight loss and health, a good, 30-minute (minimum) brisk walk, five to seven times a week, will accomplish what you need to activate your metabolism, increase circulation, and detoxify metabolic wastes.

Remember that upper-body exercise is as important as lower-body. When the arms move, the lymphatic fluid circulates around every cell. When walking, move your arms with enthusiasm. Swimming (moving the arms through water) is a particularly good form of exercise that works both the upper and lower body. Tai Chi also exercises the whole body and is a particularly beneficial exercise as it builds vitality.

The Case For More Strenuous Exertion

Regarding fat reduction, exercise is the key to an important ally, Human Growth Hormone (HGH). In the youthful years, many people were able to lay around all day and eat. Somehow, youthful bodies get away with it. Later, though, the roll of fat around the middle develops and stays there. Why? You know the process, but let's look at this from the perspective of HGH.

Human growth hormone helps us burn fat, increase lean muscle, repair damaged tissue, increase bone density, and have better energy. Sounds like the fountain of youth. So where did your HGH go? Actually, it didn't go anywhere. Your pituitary gland still has it. The problem of middle age is that your body loses the factors that cause your pituitary to release this hormone, or it loses the sensitivity to these factors, so the released hormone is less effetive. The results are weight gain and other phenomena called "aging."

If only we could have the pituitary release more of this hormone, we would have amazing, beneficial changes in our health. Here are three things you can do right now, without drugs, to increase youthfulness via HGH:

- **Exercise** – because you work the muscles, a message is sent to the pituitary to release growth hormone for repair. Here is the case for more strenuous exercise than walking. If you really work your muscles, their natural micro-tears stimulate the signal for repair and the body responds with HGH, which stimulates the growth of new muscle fibers that add to your muscular physique and create more "fires" in which to burn fat. This is why exercise, particularly weight-resistance training, helps burn fat. As you increase your muscle mass, you increase your fat-burning potential.

- **Proper Dietary Protein** – helps maintain the insulin/glucagon balance. Excessive insulin inhibits HGH. This is one reason why excessive carbohydrates in the diet turn to fat. Once fat is stored, the excessive presence of insulin prevents HGH from building muscle mass to burn more fat.

- **Ensure A Good Night's Sleep** – Deep sleep is when the body's "elf-force," otherwise known as HGH, comes out and performs its wonders. Deep sleep is a requirement for proper healing and rejuvenation. Exercise helps you sleep.

Here we find the basic premises of living *La Buena Vida,* (The Good Life,) instead of *La Vida Loca* (The Crazy Life.) Good food, good exercise, good sleep. Throw in some good friends and good experiences and you've got a recipe for success. Perhaps it doesn't sound as intriguing as painting the town, but it is the basis for a long and productive life based on your inner fountain of youth – HGH.

So where do you go from here? First, if you are sedentary, begin walking today! Go to a park, hike and bike trail, or stroll your neighborhood, or, if you are really tough, walk the mall. To maximize your inherent HGH potentials, begin a program of weight-resistance training three times a week. These small commitments will pay you huge dividends in your health, fitness and fat-loss.

CHAPTER SEVENTEEN

Fat-Burning Nutrients: Supplements To Accelerate Weight Loss

Most of the mentally retarded babies born in America are due to the mother's drug, cigarette, or alcohol addiction or their poor eating habits where they lacked the basic vitamins and minerals needed to produce a healthy baby!
– Dr. Roger Williams

Nutritional supplements can be a powerful ally in activating, accelerating, and simplifying the fat-burning processes and, thus, can play an important role in helping you lose body fat. In addition to your eating plan, which will get the job done in and of itself, the use of certain supplements can often help get the job done sooner and more efficiently. Most people need all the help they can get!

Supplements can become expensive and we don't really know in advance if they will work for us. Therefore, we want to pick the most important, most effective ones. Here is a brief discussion of supplements that can enhance your fat-weight loss goals.

Multi-Vitamin, Multi-Mineral, Multi-Antioxidants

It is of critical importance that you not have nutrient deficiencies during your fat-burning program. Since the typical person

Absolutely essential! Increase your nutrition and protect your health with a comprehensive supplement.

today falls into the category "overfed but undernourished," supplementation of daily nutrients has become the cornerstone of dietary health.

The old discussion of "Can't I get all my nutrients from my food the way Nature intended?" has become a moot point. The answer is, "No, not really." I was as reluctant as anyone to admit that we have entered an era of supplementation or "food in a pill." It goes against my core beliefs, but the evidence to supplement is overwhelming. The only solution to not supplementing is to own a 40-acre, organic farm and work it. Since I don't have the farm or the expertise, in 1989 I finally acquiesced and began supplementation to the overall improvement of my health.

12 Reasons Nutritional Supplementation is Essential

1. Nutrient-depleted soil – if the minerals are not in the soil, the plant is deficient, as are the animals and people who eat the plant.
2. Commercial, chemical fertilizers – only replace two or three minerals out of forty-four vital minerals.
3. Foods are picked green and do not ripen on the vine, bush, or tree. Their nutrients are immature and less viable.
4. Produce is stored and transported long distances. It's not fresh, which causes vitamin loss.
5. Pesticides, fungicides, and algaecides, tax our detoxification processes, thus depleting nutrients.
6. Air pollution presents a challenge to our nutrient-dependent detoxification pathways.

7. Tap water contains hundreds of chemicals, some carcinogenic.

8. Chemical preservatives and food additives contribute to the body's toxic burden.

9. Processing of food removes valuable essential fatty acids, vitamins, and minerals.

10. Prescription medications interfere with the body's chemistry and deplete nutrients.

11. Cooking destroys nutrients. We often eat too many all-cooked "fast food" meals.

12. Stress, life in the fast lane, and running the rat race demand more nutrition.

It's clear, we've got to supplement just to keep up.

Ideal Health Systems, Inc., the same company that markets the FitTest, also markets a test called the PrivaTest™. PrivaTest is used to custom-design a 55-ingredient, daily supplement called Custom Essentials™, based on laboratory analysis of urinary metabolic by-products. Again, Ideal Health Systems has provided sophisticated laboratory testing at a reduced price, along with cutting edge analysis, to produce a supplement that has the individually-determined correct amount of nutrients (vitamins, minerals, amino acids, trace minerals, anti-oxidants, super nutrients) in an organically-grown food base.

For more information about ordering a PrivaTest, contact Ideal Health Systems directly at 1-800-768-7667.

Earlier in this book, I told the story of the marathon runner from Australia. Here's the rest of his story. We left him improving his time with the stamina to run a good race – all 26.2 miles. So how did he do in the race? Well, he was unable to finish! He was disappointed, to say the least. Actually, he was very upset. He came to me in an emotional crisis. He felt singled out for Divine wrath. At first, I couldn't figure out the reason for his lack of stamina, so I asked him to write down everything he was putting into his body. Then the answer became clear.

In addition to all the good foods and supplements I had suggested for him, he was taking, on his own, a *huge* dose of anti-oxidant nutrients – Vitamins A, B complex, C, and E; *as well as* selenium *plus* high doses of grapeseed extract, high doses of pycnogenol, high doses of designer anti-oxidants such as alpha lipoic acid, coenzyme Q-10, *in addition to* herbal antioxidants such as gingko, cat's claw, green tea, and silymarin. He had read that athletes need anti-oxidant nutrients. Thus, he concluded, logically but erroneously, that as a top athlete, he must really need a lot.

What happened to him? He had overdosed on these generally good, beneficial nutrients. Metabolically, he inhibited his Citric Acid Cycle, also called Kreb's Cycle (the biochemical process where the body turns food into energy). He did not know that, when the body gets *too many anti-oxidants* the overdose can interfere with metabolic balance and the body will labor to make them pro-oxidant to try to regain balance. My recommendation was to stop the anti-oxidants. Within a week he could run the course. Soon after we figured his problem out, he left Austin to pursue marathons in other cities.

The point here is this; doesn't it make sense to find out what nutrients you really need to supplement before you start supplementing?

L-Carnitine

L-Carnitine is an amino acid that is particularly helpful for weight loss when exercise is included in the program. Its role in fat-reduction is to transport fat across the cell membranes to the mitrochondria, the cellular body that burns fat for energy. When L-Carnitine is included, some researchers think that it helps the body burn more fat and less glucose during exercise. Many research studies have been done and the results are inconclusive, so there are probably other factors that assist this process. In my clinical opinion, L-Carnitine works well when it is taken in conjunction with cardiovascular exercise, and the exercise regimen occurs twice a day. In this capacity, L-Carnitine has helped many people toward their goal of fat loss. The therapeutic dose is 4000 mg., best taken prior to a cardiovascular exercise.

Chromium Picolinate and Polynicotinate

Chromium is a trace mineral needed for glucose metabolism. It is widely used to assist weight loss programs because it helps many people reduce sugar cravings, improve energy, control the appetite, and increase muscle growth to have more cells to burn more fat. As a trace mineral, there is the possibility of taking too much, so please do not apply the "more is better" mentality. The safe and therapeutic dose is 250 mcg. with each meal (i.e.,three or four times a day.)

Chromium helps burn fat fast while preserving lean muscle mass.

Gymneme Sylvestre

The East Indian herb, *Gymneme sylvestre*, is very important for insulin-resistant and pre-diabetic people because it helps repair the pancreas' beta cells that produce insulin and helps to lower

Gymneme Sylvestre—An herbal answer to insulin/glucose imbalance as well as pancreas repair.

elevated blood glucose. As a fat-weight loss tool, Gymneme sylvestre also helps increase the cells' sensitivity to insulin, allowing less insulin to be used to accomplish blood sugar balance. This means that there is less opportunity for fat storage. The history of this herb shows it has performed when all else has failed. Thus it is a very helpful for weight loss, especially when insulin resistance is a factor. The therapeutic dose is 400 mg., three times a day, or as it occurs in combination formulas.

Pancreatic Enzymes and Bromelain

Pancreatic enzyme supplement (Pancreatin) helps decrease food intake in overeaters by stimulating appetite suppressant compounds. Per our discussion on digestion, most people need help digesting their food so their bodies can derive more nutrition. Thus, a digestive enzyme supplement can be an important part of any nutritional program. Pancreatic enzymes are important in maintaining the digestive tract by helping prevent parasites. The therapeutic dose is 750 mg of 10X pancreatin with each meal.

Bromelain is a proteolytic enzyme, meaning that it digests protein. Like pancreatin, it helps with digestion and management of the bowel. Bromelain is also known to have an anti-inflammatory action. Pineapple is the most common source of this enzyme.

Vanadium (Vanadyl Sulphate)

The trace mineral, *Vanadium*, chelated into a product called *vanadyl sulphate* has been shown to lower insulin levels, help reduce insulin resistance, and increase glycogen storage. Much of the research on this compound has been conducted on diabetics to help stabilize the dosage of insulin by injection. As a supplement, vanadyl can help people who are insulin resistant with hyperinsulemia. If used in excessive doses, there are side effects, as there are with taking any trace mineral in high amounts. The therapeutic dose is 10 mg. before each meal.

Dietary Fiber

Fiber is a terrific ally in fat-weight loss programs. It increases the time it takes for macro-nutrients (especially sugars and fats) to be absorbed into the bloodstream. Thus, fiber helps control the insulin response and the amount of fat assimilated. It also helps reduce appetite and provides a sense of fullness that helps people be more comfortable when they modify their diets to smaller portions of food. The benefits of fiber on the intestines are well-known. It cleans the bowel of unwanted mucoid matter and debris, helps build an environment for the beneficial flora, and thus supports the immune system and helps prevent cancer.

Fiber is your first-line detoxification agent.

Due to the commercial processing of foods, most fiber is discarded and removed from our diets. This has prompted many people to add fiber to their diets to overcome constipation. Lately, with fiber's reputation as a supplement that lowers cholesterol, it has become very popular. The therapeutic dose is 5 grams three times daily, with meals.

Conjugated Linoleic Acid

From our discussion on Essential Fatty Acids, we learned about linoleic acid. *Conjugated Linoleic Acid (CLA)* is a new tool in clinical nutrition. Based on the known dietary deficiency, coupled with CLA's ability to limit the effectiveness of the fat-storing enzyme, *lipoprotein lipase*, this nutrient can accelerate fat loss considerably. Researchers are optimistic that CLA also functions to help enhance muscle building in the cycle of tearing down muscles during exercise and rebuilding during rest. The therapeutic dose is 1800 mg., five times a day.

Thermogenic herbs: Cayenne and Ginger

The herbs *Cayenne (red pepper)* and *Ginger* are know as "heating" herbs in that they promote circulation and stimulate the metabolism. These herbs are often used in combination to increase the basal metabolic rate and, thus, cause the body to burn more fuel. With the diet steering the body to burn fat, cayenne and ginger increase that consumption and help the fat burn more quickly.

Choline and Inositol

Choline and *Inositol* are B-vitamins called *phospholipids* that work with fats. They are constituents of lecithin and their primary function in the body is to emulsify or disperse fat. When burning fat for energy, fat is released into the blood stream. Choline and inositol help keep it thin and flowing. These vitamins help in the processing of fat by the liver and provide a supportive role to the fat-burning process. Nutritionists often recommend talking 1200 units of lecithin containing 600 units each of Choline and Inositol, three times a day with meals.

Garcinia cambogia

The berry of the Garcinia cambogia tree contains hydroxycitric acid, a nutrient that helps burn fat several ways. First, it can help block the conversion of excessive calories to fat. It inhibits

The Asian berry that prevents the conversion of calories to fat.

an enzyme, *ATP-citratelyase*, that the body uses to convert food-calories to fat. It also increases the body's ability to store carbohydrates as glycogen, the concentrated quick-energy fuel. This helps lower the appetite because the body knows it has "money in the bank" regarding its survival fuel. This slowing down of the fat-storage mechanism helps people when their diet strays to the high carbohydrate mode. Herbs are often provided in tablet or capsule. Follow directions on the label.

Carbohydrates sneak into our diets in the form of hidden sugars. For example: I quit drinking soft drinks 20 years ago, but I had been using a drink that was nothing more than 67% fruit juice and carbonated water for those times when a sparkling beverage was enjoyable. I was shocked to find that it contained 34 grams of carbohydrate. A sugar-laden commercial soda drink contains 40 grams. I quickly switched to pure cranberry juice, diluted with water, and sweetened with stevia. My new drink has only 6 grams of carbohydrate. What a difference!

Calcium Pyruvate

Well researched for its athletic-endurance applications, *calcium pyruvate* helps the body burn fat. Taken throughout the day, pyruvate has passed scrutiny of numerous studies that show it to have a gentle effectiveness in accelerating fat loss. It works best when in conjunction with a consistent exercise regimen. The therapeutic dose is 30 grams, three times a day.

Alpha Lipoic Acid

Most commonly known for its anti-oxidant properties and ability to recycle anti-oxidant nutrients, alpha lipoic acid also figures into the

Citric Acid Cycle (Kreb's Cycle) of deriving energy from food. Research on this nutrient has shown that it stabilizes blood sugar, and thus, many diabetics have been able to reduce insulin by supplementing it into their diets. This blood sugar stability factor is helpful for people who want to trim fat from their bodies. Further, the antioxidant effect helps protect the body from oxidation of fats into damaging free radicals. The therapeutic dose is 4 mg., twice a day.

Omega-3 Essential Fatty Acids

Because most people are deficient in the Omega 3 fatty acids, and because these fatty acids are needed metabolically to keep the fat burning mechanism operative, many people supplement with an essential fatty acid formula. Often this type of supplement contains 1000 mg of omega-3 three fatty acids plus marine lipids (EPA, DHA), plus some omega-6 essential fatty acids. These different designations of fatty acids refer to the structure of the molecule. But for our purposes, an essential fatty acid supplement that is strong in the omega-3 category is most excellent, both for health and to keep the fat-burning pump primed. Therapeutic dose is 1000 to 2000 mg. per day.

What to take?

People often ask, " What is the most important supplement to take? I can't afford to take them all!" Generally, the first priority is to take a custom-designed multi-vitamin, multi-mineral, multi-antioxidant such as the Custom Essentials supplement based on laboratory testing. Additionally, the herbs Gymneme sylvestre and Garcenia cambogia make a great combination, because they accelerate fat loss, reduce sugar in the blood and help rebuild the pancreas. Also, various products are available, marketed as weight-loss aids, that contain combinations of many of the nutrients mentioned in this chapter.

CHAPTER EIGHTEEN

Meals That Heal: Ideal For Fat-Burning Weight Loss

Leave thy drugs in the chemist's pot if thou canst heal the patient with food.
- Hippocrates

Here are four recipes to get your creative side going. If you love to prepare delicious meals, you'll invent hundreds of variations from these basic ideas. If you hate to cook, all you have to do is follow the recipes. Make them up in advance and you'll have several days of mix and match variety eating.

You can easily modify these meals to accommodate your individualized *The Weight Is Over* program based on your FitTest results. The ingredients can be increased or decreased to fit your particular *The Weight Is Over* program requirements. Just increase a key macro-nutrient to fit your particular profile, and the others will automatically fall into place.

These following items can appear with any recipes, and serve as powerful ShiftRight elements to any meal. They increase the nutritional value of every meal.

Soaked seeds provide wonderful raw protein and beneficial fatty acids. The soaking softens the seeds and makes them swell up for better chewing and digestibility. Simply put two tablespoons of the hulled seed mix of sunflower seeds, sesame seeds, pumpkin seeds (as well as a couple of almonds for variety) in a glass of water. Discard the floaters (they are rancid) and let the seeds soak overnight. In the morning they are ready to use. Just drain off the water and you have a moist, plump, crunchy, raw, vegetarian, delicious fat-and-protein-enhancing super food.

Oscar salad - any mixture of raw vegetables run through a food processor. Great way to use broccoli stalks, kale, leeks, chard, cabbage, beet leaf, celery stalks, etc. After chopping, add extra ingredients such as seeds, olives, pickles, marinated artichoke hearts, etc., for varied tastes. Children often like this much better than a plain vegetable sitting on the plate. The combination of flavors is often well received, much more than a single vegetable. Somehow the mixture creates a new flavor as each vegetable enhances the flavor. Add a squeeze of lemon juice for a tangy surprise.

Sprout mixture of sunflower, alfalfa, mung, and chia sprouts. Go heavy with the sunflower sprouts and cut them into short pieces with scissors to make them easier to eat.

With these foods prepared in advance, terrific, nutritious meals can be assembled very quickly.

Breakfast Burrito

Ingredients:

(Prepare the night before and keep in storage containers.)

4 oz. fajita chicken (free range or non-hormone), marinated, cooked, and chopped
2 Tbs. soaked seeds (sunflower, pumpkin, sesame, pine nuts)
1 organic corn tortilla or 1 organic whole wheat chapati tortilla (use thin tortillas)
3 sliced olives, green or black
1 oz. grated low fat, organic Monterey jack cheese, or crumbled feta cheese
4 oz. crispy salad – organic bok choy, celery, jicama, field greens, lettuce, bell pepper
1 Tbs. olive oil (extra virgin), herb and lemon juice dressing
1 oz. chopped sunflower sprouts
3 Tbs. picante sauce or mild enchilada-type sauce
6 green beans (or vegetable medley)
1 pinch kelp powder (sprinkle in burrito)

Lay out tortilla on a plate. Place fajita chicken in a stripe down the center of the tortilla. Warm in oven. Then add soaked seeds, olives, cheese, picante sauce, a sprinkle of kelp and chopped sunflower sprouts. Roll up the tortilla.

Place green beans (or vegetable medley) in a steamer and steam for 1 minute. Keep crisp.

Serve crispy salad with olive oil/lemon juice dressing.

Vegetarian Option: Use sautéed tofu in place of chicken. For variety, smear some black beans (cooked in a crock pot without boiling to maximize the protein availability) on the tortilla. Increase the ounces of tofu and seeds to increase the protein values.

Variations are endless. Here are a few suggestions to start you thinking:

- Use different proteins in the burrito (shrimp, salmon, scallops, turkey, natural chicken hot dog, tempeh, etc.)
- Use different vegetables in the salad.
- Steam a medley of vegetables.
- Use different salad dressings, including flaxseed oil and other beneficial oils.

This wonderful *The Weight Is Over* meal provides a full spectrum of essential nutrients, balanced to ensure good digestion and support optimal health and athletic performance! The meal includes:

- carbohydrate (salad, green beans, tortilla);
- protein (chicken, seeds, cheese, sprouts);
- beneficial fatty acids (seeds, olive oil, olives, chicken, cheese);
- nucleic acids (sprouts, green beans);
- enzymes (salad, sprouts, seeds);
- fiber (seeds and vegetables); and
- a full array of vitamins, and minerals such as calcium and vital trace minerals (kelp)

This is a ShiftRight meal that meets the requirements of the *Eating Energy* 12 Optimal Nutritional Factors and supports your *The Weight Is Over* Program.

Eggs Oscar

Ingredients:
(Prepare Oscar Salad the night before and keep in a storage container.)

1 yard egg, poached
2 Tbs. soaked seeds (sunflower, pumpkin, sesame, pine nuts)
1 organic corn tortilla, or 1 organic whole wheat chapati tortilla (use thin tortillas)
3 sliced olives, green or black
1 oz. crumbled feta cheese
4 oz. Oscar Salad - an assortment of organic cabbage, bok choy, sprout mixture. celery, jicama, chives, bell pepper, parsley, cucumber, and green leafy and garden vegetables
1 Tbs. grapeseed oil, flaxseed oil, and lemon juice and ginger dressing
3 asparagus (organic), lightly steamed
1 pinch kelp powder

Lay out tortilla flat on a plate. Warm in oven. Put a yard egg in a poacher cup. To the egg white area add (poke in) chunks of feta cheese, and other surprises such as capers, pine nuts, olive slices, tomato, jalapenos, seeds, etc. Steam egg to the desired consistency.

Place asparagus in a steamer and steam for 1 minute. Keep crisp.

Assemble: Spread Oscar Salad in a circle around the edge of the tortilla. Add salad dressing to the salad. Place egg in center. Garnish with kelp powder. Serve asparagus on the side.

Vegetarian Option: Use sautéed tempeh, or veggie-seed burger in place of the egg.

Variations are endless. Here are a few suggestions to start you thinking:

- Use different vegetables in the salad.
- Use different salad dressings.
- Put a natural hollandaise sauce over the egg.

This terrific *The Weight Is Over* meal provides a full spectrum of essential nutrients, balanced to ensure good digestion and support optimal health and athletic performance! The meal includes:

- carbohydrate (salad, asparagus, tortilla);
- protein (egg, seeds, feta cheese, sprouts);

- beneficial fatty acids (seeds, grapeseed oil, flaxseed oil, olives, egg, cheese);
- nucleic acids (sprouts, asparagus);
- enzymes (salad, sprouts, seeds);
- fiber (seeds and vegetables); and
- a full array of vitamins, and minerals and vital trace minerals (kelp.)

This is a ShiftRight meal that meets the requirements of the *Eating Energy* 12 Optimal Nutrition Factors and supports your *The Weight Is Over* program.

Salmon Almondine

Ingredients:
(Prepare components the night before and keep in storage containers.)

3 to 4 oz. fresh salmon fillet
2 Tbs. soaked seeds (sunflower, pumpkin, sesame, pine nuts)
1 dollop guacamole or wedge of avocado
1 oz. grated parmesan cheese
1/2 cup Caesar salad - organic romaine lettuce, with garden vegetables with sunflower sprouts, sprinkle parmesan cheese to taste.
1 Tbs. olive oil (extra virgin) and rosemary/basil dressing for salad
1/2 cup broccoli/cauliflower (organic), lightly steamed
1 pinch kelp powder
1 oz. almond slices
1 Tbs. each – capers, lemon, rosemary
4 croutons
2 Tbs. Caesar dressing

Steam salmon in stainless steel steamer. Later, add broccoli and cauliflower to steamer so all three are ready together. Use broccoli stalks, chopped into wheels. When steamed, remove salmon skin before serving.

Prepare Caesar salad by adding chopped sunflower sprouts and an assortment of vegetables. Garnish with croutons, kelp powder and seed mix. Add salad dressing.

Sprinkle parmesan cheese over steamed vegetables and the salad. Use guacamole as a dip for the vegetables or add a slice of avocado. Sprinkle capers and almond slices over salmon, then add a squeeze of fresh lemon and rosemary.

Vegetarian Option: Use sautéed tofu, tempeh, or veggie-seed burger in place of salmon.

Variations are endless. Here are a few suggestions to start you thinking:

- Use different vegetables in the salad.
- Use different vegetables in steamer.
- Use different salad dressings.
- Put a natural lemon, caper, rosemary sauce over the salmon.

This delicious *The Weight Is Over* meal provides a full spectrum of essential nutrients, balanced to ensure good digestion and support optimal health and athletic performance! The meal includes:

- carbohydrate (salad, vegetables, croutons);
- protein (salmon, seeds, parmesan cheese, almonds,);
- beneficial fatty acids (seeds, avocado, cheese);
- nucleic acids (sprouts, broccoli, cauliflower);
- enzymes (salad, sprouts, seeds);
- fiber (seeds and vegetables); and
- a full array of vitamins, and minerals, and vital trace minerals (kelp.)

This ShiftRight meal meets the requirements of the *Eating Energy* 12 Optimal Nutrition Factors and supports your *The Weight Is Over* program.

Thai Spring Rolls

Grab one and hop in the car. You're off for a well-nourished day.

Ingredients (prepared the night before):

4 oz. chicken breast (free range or non-hormone), marinated (in ginger, or your favorite marinade), cooked, and chopped
2 Tbs. soaked seeds (sunflower, pumpkin, sesame, pine nuts)
1 spring roll wrapper or rice paper wrapper
4 sliced olives, green or black

6 oz. chopped vegetables of choice – organic bok choy, celery, jicama, cucumber, bell pepper, scallion, broccoli, snow peas, leaf lettuce
1 Tbs. olive oil (extra virgin) and lemon juice dressing or natural peanut sauce
1 oz. chopped sunflower sprouts
Optional garnishes: chopped parsley, herbs, scallions, seaweed
1 pinch kelp powder

Prepare egg-roll wrapper by package directions. Lay out the wrapper on a plate. Place chopped vegetables on the wrapper. Add ginger chicken and garnishes. Then add soaked seeds, olives, sprouts, kelp powder, and garnishes. Roll up the wrapper. These bundles of vegetables with spicy chicken bits are ready to go. Dip in a sauce of your choice.

Vegetarian Options: Use sautéed tofu or tempeh in place of chicken. For variety, add sprouted beans.

Variations are endless. Here are a few suggestions to start you thinking:

- Use different proteins in the spring roll (shrimp, salmon, scallops, crab.)
- Use different vegetables in the wrapper.
- Use different dipping sauces for wonderful variety.

This delicious *The Weight Is Over* meal provides a full spectrum of essential nutrients, balanced to ensure good digestion and support optimal health and athletic performance! The meal includes:

- carbohydrate (wrapper, vegetables);
- protein (chicken, seeds, sprouts);
- beneficial fatty acids (seeds, dipping sauce);
- nucleic acids (sprouts, vegetables);
- enzymes (vegetables, sprouts, seeds);
- fiber (seeds and vegetables); and
- a full array of vitamins, and minerals, and vital trace minerals (kelp.)

This ShiftRight meal meets the requirements of the *Eating Energy* 12 Optimal Nutrition Factors and supports your *The Weight Is Over* program.

Summary

Here we have established a new foundation for our nutritional health. All these recipes contain super nutritious foods that can help your entire diet ShiftRight into a more optimal dimension. By creating and having these foods on hand, you can upgrade your diet every time you eat.

The Breakfast Burrito and the Thai Spring Roll travel well since they are rolled up. They make a quick breakfast and can be taken to work for a fat-burning lunch.

The next chapter provides 42 meal ideas that you can follow while you are learning to focus on foods that not only prime your fat-burning mechanism but also increase your nutritional health.

CHAPTER NINETEEN

The Weight Is Over Two Week Menus

Unless we eat food properly prepared, we suffer from inferior physical development, mental instability, low endurance, and lack of resistance to infection.
- Dr. E.V. McCollum, Johns Hopkins

The following two-week plan of *The Weight Is Over* menus will help you get started and demonstrate that this program is easy to follow. A food plan should be expansive in its variety to offer a broad range of enzymes, vitamins, minerals, amino acids, fiber, essential fatty acids, and so forth. Many wonderful new foods are just waiting for you to discover them. This two-week plan will help you start now, while you are waiting for your FitTest results. Then you will find you can easily tailor these meals to fit your individual plan.

Note to *Pro-Vita! Plan* devotees accustomed to light, no protein dining at night, here we are using proteins later in the day to keep the fat-burning mechanism active via the glucagon response. This is a therapeutic approach to hormone management via diet.

Week One

	BREAKFAST	LUNCH	SUPPER
MONDAY	steamed broccoli sautéed chicken, top w/ Parmesan salad w/sprouts, soaked seeds feta & olives	steamed asparagus garlic sautéed shrimp salad w/cottage cheese soaked seeds	sautéed Chinese greens (bok choy) grilled salmon steamed 1/4 sweet potato, small salad with flaxseed oil dressing
TUESDAY	spinach omelet w/fresh salsa grated raw milk cheese salad w/sprouts soaked seeds	steamed green beans fish (orange roughie) topped w/ Parmesan salad w/ sprouts	veggie sticks w/tahini scallops marinara spelt pasta (small side dish) topped w/ parsley or cilantro
WEDNESDAY	snowpeas squid or fish salad w/sprouts, seeds, feta, veggie sticks & salsa	sautéed cabbage herb seasoned tofu salad w/sprouts, seeds, tahini dressing	garden salad turkey w/garnishes black beans w/salsa cottage cheese
THURSDAY	steamed cauliflower turkey bacon Chinese peas sprouts & seeds	green salad w/sprouts soaked seeds chicken taco w/salsa & grated raw milk cheddar	green salad, olives seafood soup veggie-seed patty w/sprouts in pita w/tofu mayo
FRIDAY	lettuce, sprouts, cottage cheese topped w/poached egg, salsa veggie sticks & tahini	sautéed green & yellow squash w/buffalo burger salad w/sprouts, seeds & feta	steamed vegetable medley Cornish game hen sprouts, garden salad w/flaxseed oil
SATURDAY	steamed broccoli garlic shrimp salad w/sprouts, seeds, feta, & olives	steamed artichoke sautéed chicken salad w/sprouts, seeds, veggie sticks & tahini	vegetables; salad shrimp kabob baked chips & salsa avocado slice
SUNDAY	broccoli omelet w/salsa grated raw milk cheddar veggie sticks & tahini	steamed asparagus w/roasted turkey breast salad w/sprouts, seeds, cottage cheese	lima beans mussels marinara mixed greens salad w/dressing

Week Two

	BREAKFAST	LUNCH	SUPPER
MONDAY	steamed broccoli & cauliflower parmesan fish or shrimp salad w/sprouts, seeds veggie sticks & tahini	sautéed carrots & snow peas spicy sesame chicken strips salad w/ sprouts, seeds cottage cheese	sautéed greens barbecue chicken baked chips & salsa Caesar salad
TUESDAY	scrambled eggs w/sprouts in taco w/salsa & feta cheese, olives veggie sticks & salsa	Brussels sprouts miso-fish soup salad w/sprouts, seeds, cottage cheese	garden salad ground chicken tacos guacamole (avocado, tomato, garlic, spices)
WEDNESDAY	steamed green beans scrambled herbed tofu salad w/sprouts, seeds, feta, olives	steamed asparagus BBQ shrimp salad w/seeds, sprouts, cottage cheese	stir fry: snow peas, bok choy, w/ daicon radish, water chestnuts, ginger chicken cucumber salad
THURSDAY	sautéed cabbage steamed chicken breast w/grated raw milk cheddar salad w/seeds, sprouts, raisins	sautéed Chinese greens garlic sautéed squid or fish w/Parmesan; salad w/seeds, sprouts, feta	steamed cabbage buffalo burger patty, black-eyed peas field green salad
FRIDAY	steamed broccoli chicken fajitas, feta veggie sticks, olives	vegetable medley seafood stew salad w/sprouts, seeds	asparagus with sauce broiled herbed fish filet Caesar salad
SATURDAY	sautéed snow peas chicken taco w/sprouts, salsa, & grated cheese veggie sticks w/tahini	steamed green beans or greens w/garlic shrimp cashews field green salad w/dressing	vegetable soup king crab w/lemon vegetable medley salad w/dressing
SUNDAY	sautéed vegetables, basil/herb omelet salad w/seeds, sprouts	vegetable medley roasted chicken breast cucumber salad	garden Salad chicken & vegetable soup stuffed olives

To further your skills, here is more discussion. This information is for people who want to optimize their nutritional intake while losing weight. This detailed approach takes planning, but like many things in life, the rewards are greater because of the planning.

How To Construct The Optimal Meal

Let's see what a well-thought-out meal (one that maximizes proteins and minimize stress and toxins) might be. To design an optimal meal, we use five sources of protein (one cooked, four raw) and five vegetables (one cooked, four raw). The volume on the plate will be 65-75% vegetables and 25-35% low-stress protein foods, with a touch of the beautiful and good fats (salad dressing, seeds, nuts).

Composition of a 5+ 5 Eating Energy Plan Optimal Meal

Macro-nutrient Source	Preparation Method	Percentage on Plate
Low-stress proteins	1 cooked, 4 raw	25% - 35%
Vegetables	1 cooked, 4 raw	65% - 75%
Beautiful & Good Fats		a touch

This combination will provide maximum nutrition. This is called the 5+5 *Eating Energy* Plan and has helped thousands of people improve their health while losing weight.

- The five protein sources guarantee that the amino acids will be complete, and provide fatty acids.
- The five vegetables provide a variety of enzymes, chlorophyll, fiber, and chromatin factors (DNA/RNA) to buffer the protein acids and assist with digestion and assimilation.
- The vegetables also provide the optimal carbohydrates for an easily accessible energy supply, as well as some fatty acids.

- A bit of balanced, organic butter on the cooked vegetables, a little flaxseed oil on a salad, a few olives or a slice of avocado on the plate, or simply the oils found in seeds, will provide the lipid factors that will be used by the liver to humanize the protein so that it can function non-allergenically.

Do not eat starch-carbohydrates with this protein vegetable meal. This includes sugars, potatoes, rice, breads, crackers, cereals and grains.

Below is a list, divided into the 5+5 categories. This list shows numerous examples of foods you can use to construct an optimal meal.

1 cooked protein = fresh fish (cod, halibut, herring, mackerel, mahi-mahi, mullet, snapper, octopus, scallops, shrimp, squid), eggs (soft boiled, poached, scrambled), or for the vegetarian, tofu burger, tempeh, or miso soup.

4 raw proteins = soaked organic seeds (sunflower, sesame, pumpkin, squash, flaxseed, chia, pine nuts, etc.) sunflower sprouts, alfalfa sprouts, low fat or nonfat cottage cheese, French feta cheese, tahini, and a few nuts (almond, cashew, walnut, pecan, etc.).

1 cooked vegetable = broccoli, bok choy, artichoke, cauliflower, kale, collards, green beans, asparagus, cabbage, celery, green and red bell pepper, and most any of the other "pot herb" vegetables available, or a green leafy vegetable.

4 raw vegetables = salad of leaf lettuce (not iceberg), endive, spinach, arrugula, cress, dandelion, celery, tomato, cauliflower, carrot, beet, radish, jicama, parsley, cabbage, cucumber, collards, beet greens, kale, cucumber (without the skin), sprouts (they do double duty as both vegetable and protein.)

Have a great time re-designing your health and physique with your individualized *The Weight Is Over Program.*

CHAPTER TWENTY

ShiftRight Substitutions and Shopping Guide

...most of us today are suffering from certain dangerous dietary deficiencies which cannot be remedied until the depleted soils are brought into proper mineral balance...fruits and vegetables and grains now being raised on millions of acres of land that no longer contains enough of certain needed minerals are starving us no matter how much of them we eat.
- U.S. Government Document 264

Health-Nut Joe's "Fun House Ride"

Dramatization – Rod Serling appears on the TV screen. His voice, raspy from his 62nd cigarette, but, edged with compassion, states matter of factly, "This is a sad story, but one that brings a ray of hope to many. With the camera, our window to the mind's eye, we'll accompany Health-Nut Joe in a re-enactment of his famous visit to the grocery store. All else aside, this promises to be an historic event. Not everyone goes shopping and enters [dramatic pause] The Twilight Zone."

On entering the cool, bright, color-dazzle of this "world of choices," we can't help but stare in amazement at all the selection. At no time in history have so much variety and so many choices in foods been assembled in one place. Other than plucking a low-hanging fruit from the tree, where else have so many timesaving conveniences been placed within arm's-reach for the human race? Surely this must be heaven or at least a pinnacle of human achievement. What good fortune that we live in such technologically-advanced times where we can enjoy so much of the Earth's bounty.

Like a person with a guidebook to Disney World, Health-Nut Joe begins a systematic and thorough shopping experience. He chooses a shopping cart with an eccentric wheel and moves quickly down the first aisle, barely glancing at the row upon row of laxatives, antacids, antiperspirants, antibiotic creams, hemorrhoid preparations, enema bags, and drugs to relieve pain. He looks a little disappointed and perplexed, but smiles when he rounds the corner into the refrigerated dairy section.

Soon he has a fearful look in his eyes. He reads labels and puts products back on the shelf. "This milk has been pasteurized (destroyed enzymes), homogenized (altered fats) and has synthetic Vitamin D, and antibiotic residue," he moans, "and all this cheese, too." In disgust, he turns quickly and heads down the aisle, saying something about the margarine containing partially-hydrogenated oils that cause cardiovascular disease."

"Yikes!" he screams. He's heading down the aisle of soda pop. He moves to the center of the aisle lest one grab him from the shelf and pour caffeine, sugar, preservatives, aspartame, phosphoric acid, and chemicals down his throat. He controls his hallucination and hesitates. There on the lower shelf is a bottle of spring water. He reaches for it, and cries out in disgust, "It is just filtered tap water with minerals added!" He grabs a bottle of a French water claiming "bottled at the source," and rounds the next aisle, cruising past the display rack of rancid oil-fried corn chips with preservatives and artificial flavors without even glancing at their beckoning, plump bags. He's on his fourth aisle, but feels a little more secure having at least one product in his cart.

He moves swiftly past the processed flour cake mixes and processed grain, sugar-laden cereals, almost running for the meat market at the end of the aisle. The wheel on his cart flips around sideways, making a clacking sound. He searches frantically for a non-hormoned, non-force-fattened meat. There is none. Controlling his panic, he spies a salmon filet. He asks the fish market employee, "Can you guarantee this fish has not been treated with sulfites?" With the affirmative reply, and with a little more assurance, he adds the salmon filet to his cart containing a bottle of water.

The next aisle features motor oil, anti-freeze, and further down, bottles of cooking oil. "Whoa," exclaims Joe, "That'll kill you. Look at all this heat-altered, processed, polyunsaturated oil, and, oh dear, here's the shortening." He picks up the can of shortening and muses, "Lard would be better than this. I'll take saturated fat over partially-hydrogenated fat any day." His hand shakes as he sets the can back on the shelf, but the can wobbles, then crashes to the floor. Joe is too far-gone to notice.

His eyes get a glazed look. Row upon row of canned goods beckon. He searches labels quickly, "Sugar, sugar, preservatives, sugar, chemicals, sugar, partially-hydrogenated fats, preservatives," he chants, putting each can back. "Cooked to death," he moans and heads for the next aisle. "Dead, dead, they're all dead," he moans in liturgy.

Here reside the condiments. Joe adds a bottle of Tabasco to his cart and a jar of pimento. Obviously, he's thrilled that he found something to put in the cart. He quickly clears three remaining aisles of refined flour products, candy, jellies, syrups, and sugar without so much as an anxious glance. He hesitates at the end of aisle 17, just past the bug sprays and repellants, and takes a step to bolt screaming for the door. Something green catches his eye. There, like a beacon in the dark night of soul, he sees the haven of the produce department. Bin upon bin of fruits and vegetables await him.

Tentatively, he takes his first step, then another and another. The cart wheel clicks merrily as the cart crabs sideways. He abandons the cart and runs, arms outstretched for the vegetable display. As he rushes up, the sprinklers come and soak his arms, but that doesn't daunt him. He's found home.

"Aaaaaaggggggghhhhhhh!" he cries out. The pain is unbearable. "These vegetables are grown with synthetic fertilizer in impoverished soil and sprayed with pesticides!" He falls to the floor thrashing his legs. Known for his perseverance, he pulls himself up. Clawing at the edge of the bins, he scoots over to the fruit section.

"Aaaaaaggggghhhhh!" he cries again. These fruit were picked green and force-ripened with chemicals. They've been sprayed with numerous pesticides and the watermelons were grown in Mexico with the DDT that the US banned years ago (and sent to Mexico) and fertilized with Hitler's nerve-gas stores from World War Two. Dizzily, he walks around in circles, muttering to himself.

Realizing that intervention was necessary, Rod Serling took Joe's arm, now weakened and shaking with fright. "Here, Joe," he consoled. "Here is the organic produce bin." He stood him in front of a small bin of molding lemons and flowering broccoli, noting that the prices were double compared to the other bins. "Take this organic orange, and go sit outside. I'll check out and take you home."

The camera zooms in on Rod Serling's face. "Everyone has their secret fright in the dark recesses of their psyche. For some, it's being mauled by a dinosaur. For others it's being the only person alive on Earth. For Health-Nut Joe, it's lies near the surface in the mundane experience of grocery shopping. But for every person walking this planet, look left, look right, you're only a heartbeat away from [dramatic pause] The Twilight Zone.

Substitutions: Choose Life Over Death, Health Over Disease

It was a rough and rude awakening for Health Nut Joe. However, he recovered well with the help of the Natural Foods Store a mile from his home. A week later, over a cup of herbal tea and a lovely sprout salad, I visited with Joe about his wild adventure that he compared to Dante's *Inferno*. "You see," he said, "it's really just a matter of substitutions. All we really have to do to our diets is ShiftRight – delete some of the really detrimental foods we are eating and add some the really terrific foods – that upgrades our entire health picture, not to mention discarding a lot of useless fat in our bodies."

So here are the "bare bones" but critically important substitutions you can make right now to your diet to ShiftRight to reduce the sugars and detrimental fats so you can lose weight, enjoy alleviation of symptoms, live in a more optimal state of health. I got this list from Health Nut Joe, who by the way, cut off his ponytail and opened up a chemical-free shopping cart repair business. Shares are traded on the American Stock Exchange.

Substitutions exist on a ShiftRight continuum. Oftentimes it is difficult to jump from the left side to the right side all at once because we are often very happy with our little indiscretions and addictions. Thus, it is better to take "baby steps" in the right direction and let Nature help us move into a more healthy diet.

Here are the topmost three ShiftRight steps to improve your diet for optimal fat burning and health.

1. **Throw out refined sugar and refined sugar products.** Toss all the breakfast cereals, donuts, candy, cakes, pies, pastries, sugar-bowl, jellies, cookies, and sodas in your pantry. Don't give them to charity or the food bank.

   Substitute. Now, before you go into sugar-withdrawal shock, you can **replace** those foods with fresh fruit, and some fruit-juice-sweetened cookies from the heath food store to use judiciously in transition.

2. **Throw out partially-hydrogenated fats.** This includes shortening and shortening products, corn chips, potato chips, taco shells, white bread, margarine, pastries, and canned goods with "partially-hydrogenated" on the label. Don't give them to charity or the food bank. They are not gifts of health.

   Substitute with baked chips, grapeseed oil, whole grain bread, and foods from the health food store. Remember to read labels at the health food store because partially-hydrogenated fats turn up like weeds.

3. **Throw out refined, white-flour products.** These include white bread, biscuits, pies, cakes, pizza crusts, cookies, flour, bagels, and wheat tortillas. As you reduce these products, your self-inflicted damage to your metabolism and excessive fat-weight will diminish.

   Substitute small amounts of whole grain products, and fill your tummy with real vegetables. This is a major boost to your overall nutrition intake and removes a primary cause of fat-weight gain.

Oftentimes, a small substitution and a less-frequent use of detrimental substance will make a profound change. Here are a couple of examples.

Let's say a person has a problem with coke addiction. I'm not talking about the illegal drug from the coca plant. I'm talking about the legal "drug" called soda pop from the grocery store. Here is a step by step program for breaking free and saving your health, and reducing fat-poundage.

First, buy a soda-pop substitute from the health food store. This product will probably be caffeine-free, chemical and preservative free, and use high fructose corn sweetener rather than refined sugar. While not a paragon of virtue as it still contains phosphoric acid and a load of sweet, it does represent a small ShiftRight, a baby step in the right direction.

Now, if you were drinking four sugar-sodas a day, cut back to two of the more natural ones. This is a clear 50% reduction in soda-source sugar intake – a considerable net gain during the transition period. Just add a couple of apples or other fruit for the other two sugar-feedings you were accustomed to. Then continue to diminish gradually.

As your body adapts and appreciates the new improvements, you will be able to take the next step, which is to eliminate the whole soda thing and find joy and satisfaction in something even more healthful. Perhaps it's sparkling water with lime. Perhaps it's a floral herbal tea, maybe sweetened with stevia. Just keep moving away from sugar toward beverages that provide nutrition. When it's time for a dessert or treat, use Nature's luscious desert – fresh fruit.

Perhaps your undoing is those little chocolate donuts that helped the actor, comedian John Belushi win the decathlon. When you reach for the donut, simply earn it by eating a stalk of celery first. Then eat a stalk of celery between each donut. This will result in an increase in nutrition and fiber via the celery and a decrease in the donuts because you'll become full faster. Yet, you are not deprived of the donut experience – you simply shifted it to the right. Later, you'll be able to ditch the donuts and substitute a health food store snack, or better yet, skip the snack because you don't really need it and have no desire for it. It wasn't that good anyway.

Isn't it great to live in technological times where we have technological answer to the problems caused by technology? We have many substitutes for the empty harvest that lines the grocery store shelves. These substitutes can be found in the health food store as well as in the commercial grocery stores, since they pay homage to the dollar and demand of an increasingly aware public who wants natural foods put back into our diets.

The three ShiftRight substitution steps we just discussed will provide enormous benefits as you weed out the undoing of your health and reclaim the methods of eating that support your health and optimal weight.

ShiftRight Shopping Guide

To help you get ready for your *The Weight Is Over* adventure, here is an instant shopping list to stock the fridge with the foods that will support both fat-weight loss and overall nutritional health improvement. You can bring these items into your home now and begin using them before you get your FitTest results.

1. **Pure Water.** Buy some bottles of pure water, line 'em up, and drink 'em down. Follow the instructions in the "Water's Role in Fat Loss and Health" chapter.

2. **Vegetables.** Get a large assortment of salad fixings, organically grown if available. Lettuce, cabbage, bok choy, beet leaf, field greens, celery, sunflower sprouts, cucumber, tomatoes, scallions, etc. Also, get vegetables for steaming, such as broccoli, cauliflower, green beans, lima beans, asparagus, squash, etc. For fun, pick out a vegetable you've never had before. (OK, it may not strike you as fun, but do it for the sake of variety.) Get kohlrabi, kale, cactus, diakon, turnips, jicama, or whatever strikes your fancy. You don't know until you try.

3. **Sunflower Seeds, Sesame Seeds, Pumpkin Seeds and Pine Nuts.** Get a pound each of this great selection of seeds. You'll soak them overnight in water and sprinkle a tablespoon or two on your salad.

4. **Fresh Fruit.** Purchase an assortment of fresh fruit – apples, oranges, peaches, pears, grapes, cherries, grapefruit, and even exotic fruit such as star fruit, persimmons, kumquat, and kiwi fruit, as well as melons such as honeydew and cantaloupe. These will provide refreshment and satisfy the urge for something sweet if it occurs.

5. **Substitute Foods.** Identify the foods that you know will cause you problems if they are not available. Find a substitute to try. For example, if you love PureFat Porkbelly brand of bacon loaded with nitrates, try some low fat, preservative-free turkey bacon from the health food store. If you must have ice cream in the evening, put some grapes in the freezer and use them for a sweet, cold snack. If you have a passion for corn chips, get a bag or two of the baked, organic grain chips. Start experimenting. By checking labels, you may find that a product such as ketchup contains a lot of sugar. You may find a more natural, lower-sugar "katsup" at the health food store. Grab some.

6. **Nuts in the shell.** Pick up an assortment of nuts in the shell. Don't wait for Christmas. Use these with your meals and be sure you have a nutcracker.

With this list, you'll have natural whole foods in the pantry. Your nutrition just increased, your fat-building foods just decreased, and for many, a whole new world of tastes just opened.

CHAPTER TWENTY-ONE

Harness Your Fat Burning Power

You'll see it when you believe it.
You'll believe it when you write it.
When you write it, it's yours.
— *Lou DeCaprio*

By now, your FitTest is enroute to you. Soon your FitTest results will guide you toward your goal of fat loss as well as improved overall health. Did I say **"goal?"** You know, a goal has got to be more than wishful thinking or a general idea. A goal occurs when you can see, feel, hear, smell, taste, and know that you really are what you affirm you are. You must create your success by decree. So now, there are just a few more simple steps to take to fully realize that nothing, absolutely nothing will get in your way of becoming the person you see deep inside – fit, trim, healthy, and free to live the life of your choosing.

Checklist For Success – The Seven Simple ShiftRight Steps

Use this Checklist For Success to make certain you are absolutely, positively on the right track, non-stop to creating the physique, the health, and the life you want to live.

1. **Order your FitTest.** Also order your PrivaTest as well and build a nutritional foundation for more effective weight loss.

2. **Take your FitTest right away.** Don't delay. Procrastination is a stake in the heart. You can take your PrivaTest at the same time.

3. **Make a Shop Stop.** Use the Instant Shopping List from Chapter 20 to get you started. Pick up the vegetables and fruit and some of the ShiftRight substitutions from Chapter 20 that you are going to incorporate into your diet. Refer to the menus in Chapter 18: Meals That Heal and Chapter 19: Two Week *The Weight Is Over* Menus for more ideas.

4. **Toss out the items that will pull you down.** See the "Throw It Out" list in Chapter 20.

5. **Prepare a reward** for yourself when you reach your goal. Of course, health and fitness is its own reward, but it's fun to have a personal reward to say, "Thanks. I did it." Plan on purchasing new clothes or strutting your stuff on the beach, taking a trip, or being outspoken about this program so others can benefit. Your reward can be whatever motivates you and will be a moment of accomplishment.

6. **Complete the charts below.**

7. **Schedule some time for exercise.** Some should be *daily*, such as a walk or a swim. Some could be *three times a week*, such as weight resistance training at the gym.

Chart Your Course and Mark Your Progress

The act of writing things down harnesses a special use of your creative faculties that makes a mould for success. You use both your right brain (creative mind) and your left brain (motor skills and logic) to bring your full force of commitment to the forefront.

First, write down all the reasons you want to lose weight. Think of them all, including looking good, getting back into "those" clothes, better self-image, better health, etc.

Why I, (your name) ______________________ want to lose weight:

1. ______________________

2. ______________________

3. ______________________

4. ______________________

5. ______________________

6. ______________________

7. ______________________

Next, write down your specific goals, such as the number of pounds, or dress sizes, or belt notches, or inches – whatever is meaningful to you.

I, (your name) ______________________ will lose _____ pounds.

I, ______________________ will trim down to _____.

Next, write down your health goals. It is not uncommon that people experience the remission of symptoms such as hypoglycemia, arthritis, fibromyalgia, fatigue, headaches, low libido, pre-menstrual symptoms, constipation, and allergies. Link your nutritional work with the freedom from annoying symptoms.

I, ______________________ will benefit from the improvement of these symptoms because I increase my nutrition and allow my body to heal according to its inherent wisdom:

1. ____

2. ____

3. ____

4. ____

5. ____

6. ____

7. ____

Finally, write down your reward:

My personal reward to enjoy on the inevitable success of my program is: ______________________________

Find a picture that represents your reward and paste it on your bathroom mirror. For example, if you plan a vacation trip to an island beach, tape up a photo of the beach. Call your travel agent and make reservations because you will be there.

Now you're armed and dangerous! You have goals and the power of commitment launched by seeing them in print. You have charted your course. To mark your progress, complete this information every week.

Progress Charts:

Start Date ______________

Weight _____, Waist Measurement _____, Hip Measurement _____

Week One: Date ______________

Weight _____, Waist Measurement _____, Hip Measurement _____

Week Two: Date ______________

Weight _____, Waist Measurement _____, Hip Measurement _____

Week Three: Date ______________

Weight _____, Waist Measurement _____, Hip Measurement _____

Week Four: Date ______________

Weight _____, Waist Measurement _____, Hip Measurement _____

Week Five: Date ______________

Weight _____, Waist Measurement _____, Hip Measurement _____

Week Six: Date ______________

Weight _____, Waist Measurement _____, Hip Measurement _____

Week Seven: Date ______________

Weight _____, Waist Measurement _____, Hip Measurement _____

Week Eight: Date ___________

Weight _____, Waist Measurement _____, Hip Measurement _____

Week Nine: Date ___________

Weight _____, Waist Measurement _____, Hip Measurement _____

Week Ten: Date ___________

Weight _____, Waist Measurement _____, Hip Measurement _____

Week Eleven: Date ___________

Weight _____, Waist Measurement _____, Hip Measurement _____

Week Twelve: Date ___________

Weight _____, Waist Measurement _____, Hip Measurement _____

Week Thirteen: Date ___________

Weight _____, Waist Measurement _____, Hip Measurement _____

Week Fourteen: Date ___________

Weight _____, Waist Measurement _____, Hip Measurement _____

Week Fifteen: Date ___________

Weight _____, Waist Measurement _____, Hip Measurement _____

Week Sixteen: Date ___________

Weight _____, Waist Measurement _____, Hip Measurement _____

Share Your Success With Ideal Health®, International

Part of the joy of being the one to share this information with you is to share, in a very small way, in your success. If you'd like to communicate your success with Ideal Health, they would enjoy hearing from you. Write to:

Ideal Health, International
50 Salem Street
Lynnfield, MA 01940

Now the time has come to wrap up our time together. The next chapter features parting comments and final thoughts. When you finish this book, don't put it on the shelf or in the garage. Instead, put it on the kitchen counter so you can refer to it when you prepare meals and your shopping list. Keep this program in the forefront of your mind so the frenetic pace of life doesn't steal your dreams. Let *The Weight Is Over* be a token of inspiration when you are in your kitchen.

CHAPTER TWENTY-TWO

On Your Mark, Get Set, The Weight Is Over, Go!

Well, it's almost time for me to sign off and leave you to the success of your *The Weight Is Over* Program. I have enjoyed communicating with you and hope you've found some valuable knowledge in these pages. More than food for thought, I have aimed to provide information that will motivate you to make some simple, powerful changes in your lifestyle – ones that will bring ideal weight, optimal health, and, thus, great improvements in the quality of your life. Frankly, it is my belief that this information can revolutionize your health picture.

We've actually covered a lot of ground in a short time. As overwhelming as it may initially seem, it really boils down to the seven simple ShiftRight steps in Chapter 21's "Checklist for Success." If you do those seven steps, you'll be positioned to make the changes that really matter. Plus you'll have the power of commitment backing you up, propelling you along, helping you to achieve what you darn well know you can achieve if you simply put your mind and this plan to it!

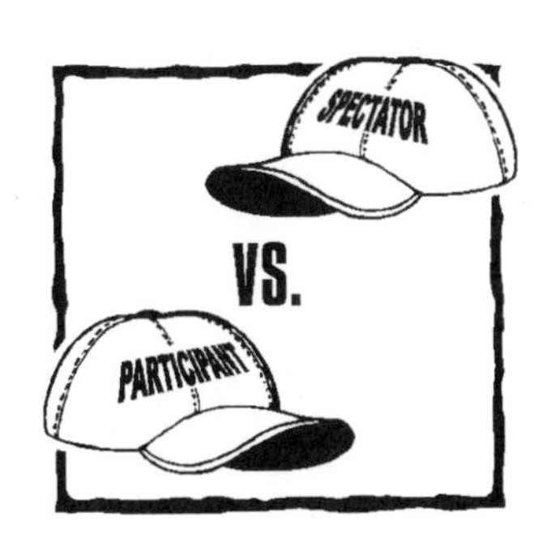

My final plea is this: did you really do the checklist, or did you keep your spectator, "I'm just a reader" hat on and turn the pages without doing the activity of harnessing your commitment for positive change? If you are still in the "just checking it out" mode, now's the time to stop and change hats. You can't be a nonchalant spectator of life and succeed. You've got to get into the ballpark and play the game to win! The *Weight Is Over* Program is a homerun. Let's check the checklist again.

Are you getting tested and allowing *The Weight Is Over* Program to work for you? Do you have a shopping list to bring home the bacon? Actually, I mean to bring home the fruits and vegetables! (Just testing you! You can bring home some bacon, too, but hopefully it's the nitrate-free health food store variety.) Are you bold and adventuresome enough to make a clean sweep and throw away the foods that are robbing you of your health and contributing to excess fat? Or do you choose a more gentle, transitional program of adding in some ShiftRight super foods and taking it a step at a time? Either way will work. You can make many small changes over a long period of time, or you can make larger changes over a shorter period of time for faster results. It's your choice. Make room in your life and pantry for foods that support your health and go get 'em!

Will you congratulate yourself with a reward? It takes a special person to acknowledge himself or herself with a truly-earned token of accomplishment. It's not really an indulgence; it's deserved. Some people need to let go and love themselves enough to do something good for themselves. Success comes as a result of the simple equation:

Belief in yourself that you can accomplish your goals

+

A plan of action

+

Acting on that plan

+

Perseverance until the goal is attained

=

Success

Finally, did you take yourself seriously enough to write down your goals? I could have said, "Did you take *this book* seriously enough to write down your goals?" but that's not really the issue, is it? I hope you don't feel I'm being too pushy. That's not my intent. The question is this: Are you ready in your life for the changes that really matter? Are you ready to create a new, more vibrant, lean body and better state of health? Or are you already indulging in self-defeating mind-talk, procrastination, fear, and slavery of staying in the same old rut? Again, I'm not pushing you, just gently nudging if you choose to let me. I just want to give you every opportunity to succeed.

Carpe Diem – Seize The Day

I propose that now is the turning point. I hope you are thrilled you read this far because the pages are running out and now is the time you can make the decision that affects your health for the rest of your life. You have the tool in your hands to participate in the most streamlined fat-loss, health-boosting, dietary plan available today.

Reach up and ask yourself if you're ready. Of course you are! So with all the decisiveness in the fibers of your being, let's get started **NOW!** Join the thousands of people who are experiencing fat loss and health improvements with *The Weight Is Over* Program.

Now for a note of inspiration. Here is an open letter from the editor of this book. She wrote this unsolicited note, with no vested interest, to communicate encouragement to you.

Dear Reader,

I'm pumped! I've just finished reading Jack's last few words as we prepare this text for the presses. I can't wait to order the FitTest and get started! Even in the midst of checking for commas and spelling, etc., I feel he's just given me the information to unlock a puzzle that's been troubling me for several years – why my weight increases or stays the same despite my attempts to do the right thing. Now I know why some foods have been tasting so good to me for quite some time – they're the ones with the healthy components he mentioned. I understand why walnuts are so yummy, and why I never seem to tire of ocean salmon, even though I don't care for the farm-raised kind. I wasn't just picky; my body was smart enough to cue me in to some healthy choices.

Now I'm motivated to start planning each meal around the lovely vegetables that I always have in my refrigerator, and am committed to not letting any of them stay there so long that they spoil! While I've been editing, I've incorporated more vegetables into our diet, and, using Jack's tips, my husband hasn't even noticed it, and has never suggested a change in the vegetables I suggest as we plan our menus. Wow! That's a minor miracle for the wife of a true meat and potatoes fan, who loves to cook, but just likes his veggies on the side! We already eat a large variety of vegetables, but I'm committed to a quest of bringing in some fun variations on a regular basis now.

I'm looking forward to stalking my pantry for the unwanted killers lurking there. Now I know what to eliminate, and why, and what I can use to replace those bad guys.

Thank goodness Jack wrote that I don't have to be perfect, and can take ShiftRight steps to correct the bad habits some "learned" diet counselors have taught me. That approach has me breathing a sigh of relief, knowing that success doesn't require perfection or immediate, huge changes.

I can't wait for the book to come off the press to reread it. (I can't believe I'm saying that; usually after working so intensely with a book, I don't want to see it again for a while!) I want to order more copies for my friends and family.

For you, I wish the same sense of empowerment and motivation that reading this text has given me.

God bless you richly,

Cathy Buettner

Conclusion

This is it. Rather than the end of this book, I boldly suggest it's a new beginning. The stakes are high in the game of life, and here, right now, you can start a fabulous program to lose excess fat and improve your health. With *The Weight Is Over* Program, you are not alone, but with the FitTest information and this book, you can quietly custom design a plan that will work and will continue to work for the "best" of your life. It's been my honor to spend this time with you. Vaya con Dios and Best Wishes In Your Health Endeavors!

Reference

The Winner's Circle

APPENDIX A

The Approximate Glycemic Index Of Selected Foods

Some carbohydrates in foods significantly stress the pancreas's insulin response and the body's blood sugar regulatory mechanism, and some carbohydrate foods are gentle and fit right into the body's energy pathways. The foods with a *high glycemic index* are often considered *high-stress foods.* There are a few exceptions of whole vegetables that rate a high index, such as carrots, beets, and parsnips, but can best be used in small amounts with other vegetables (as in a salad). Thus their glycemic index is not a significant factor because they are buffered by other foods. The foods with a low glycemic index are generally low-stress in that regard but still must meet the other *Eating Energy* 12 Optimal Food Factors to be considered a low stress food. Regarding fat-weight loss, low glycemic carbohydrate foods are the best.

Glycemic Index tables are only approximate. Variables depend on the test subjects and their predisposition to insulin responses; the actual carbohydrate, fiber, and nutrient content of a food; and whether the food is cooked or raw.

A slice of white bread sets the numeric standard with a score of 100, as it converts smoothly to glucose. All foods' numeric values on the glycemic index are relative to the effect of white bread on the secretion of insulin. It's interesting to consider a piece of refined, denatured white bread to be the same as a spoon of sugar when you are preparing a meal for children. Now, perhaps, we have a glimpse of why the dentists stay so busy filling teeth, and why we've seen such a rise in diabetes and chronic, degenerative diseases.

Fruit	Approx. Glycemic Index
Apple, red delicious	49
Apple juice	61
Apple sauce	52
Apricots	73
Bananas	84
Blackberries	24
Blueberries	26
Cherries	23
Dates	95
Grapefruit	26
Grapes	45
Kiwi fruit	38
Lemon	44
Lime	44
Mangos	78
Nectarine	28
Oranges	59
Orange juice	71
Papayas	75
Peaches	26
Pears	49
Pineapple	45
Plums	26
Prunes	52
Raisins	93
Raspberries	32

Strawberries 46

Tangerines 58

Watermelon 54

Starchy-Sugar Vegetables	Approx. Glycemic Index
Beets	64
Carrots	92
Corn	80
Parsnips	70
Potato, instant mashed	120
Potato, mashed	117
Potato, white, boiled	80
Potato, red, boiled	70
Potato, russet, baked	116
Potato, chips	77
Sweet potato	70
Yam	74

Non-Starchy Vegetables	Approx Glycemic Index
Artichoke, steamed	25
Asparagus, steamed	22
Broccoli, raw	23
Brussels Sprouts, raw	23
Cauliflower, raw	21

And many others including cabbage, celery, cucumber, endive, escarole, green beans, lettuce (all kinds), mushrooms, onion, radish, snow peas, spinach, sprouts, tomato, etc.

Nuts	Approx. Glycemic Index

All nuts have very low glycemic indexes ranging between 14 and 18.

Legumes: Peas, Beans	Approx. Glycemic Index
Beans, baked	70
Beans, garbanzo, sprouted	46
Beans, garbanzo cooked	64
Beans, kidney, dried	43
Beans, kidney, canned	71
Beans, lima	35
Beans, navy	57
Beans, pinto, dry	60
Beans, pinto, canned	65
Beans, soy, canned	20
Beans, soy, dried	22
Beans, white	54
Black-eyed peas	53
Chickpeas, sprouted	42
Chickpeas, cooked	47
Chickpeas, canned	60
Lentils, dried	36
Lentils, canned	74
Peanut	28
Peas, green, dried	50
Peas, green, frozen	65

Dairy Products	Approx. Glycemic Index
Ice cream	69
Ice cream, low fat	90
Milk (non-fat)	46
Milk (whole)	44
Yogurt, plain	52
Yogurt, frozen, fat-free	92
Yogurt, with fruit compote	68

Grains	Approx. Glycemic Index
Barley, whole pearls	36
Barley, rolled	65
Buckwheat, whole	68
Buckwheat, rolled	78
Bread, French baguette	130
Bread (French)	108
Bread (white)	100
Bread (processed whole wheat)	100
Bread (pumpernickel)	78
Bread (whole rye)	47
Corn on the cob	80
Corn, popcorn	133
Millet, whole	81
Millet, processed	103
Oats, rolled	92
Oatmeal, non processed	48
Pasta (white, boiled 15 min.)	67
Pasta (White, boiled 5 min.)	45

Pasta (whole wheat, boiled 15 min)	67
Rice (brown)	81
Rice (white)	81
Rice cakes	132
Rice, instant polished, boiled	121
Rice, polished, boiled	83
Rice (whole grain, parboiled)	54
Rye (whole grain)	47
Ryemeal	89
White Flour	100

Cereals	Approx. Glycemic Index
All Bran	74
Cornflakes	121
GrapeNuts	94
Oatmeal, instant	89
Oatmeal, whole,	50
Puffed corn	130
Puffed rice	132
Puffed wheat	110
Shredded Wheat	97

Sugar	Approx. Glycemic Index
Fructose	26
Glucose	138
Honey	126
Lactose	78
Maltose	150
Sucrose	83

Apple-A-Day Press Catalog

*Dedicated to the healing
of the whole person.*

How To Order Eating Energy!

Eating Energy is the latest in dietary nutrition and is due to be completed in March, 2000. It starts with the nutrition classic – *The Pro-Vita! Plan For Optimal Nutrition* – and launches its premises with startling new insights and in-depth Ancient Wisdom. *The Weight Is Over* is a preview of the style, simplicity, humor, and overview that brings *Eating Energy* nutrition into the 21st Century. Long awaited, *Eating Energy* simplifies your dietary dilemmas and shows how you can ShiftRight your kitchen to be your foundation of optimal health and freedom from the myriad health symptoms that plague humankind today. *Eating Energy* is destined to become the nutrition standard for optimal health in the new millennium. Learn how to master nutritional health – for yourself, and your family – and experience the priceless gift of health for the rest of your life.

Reserve your first edition now. Simply provide the following information and reserve your copy of *Eating Energy.* You will be notified as it goes to press, so you can receive it immediately, signed by the author. Send your name, address, phone number and e-mail address (if available) to Apple-A-Day Press.

In the interim, read *The Pro-Vita! Plan For Optimal Nutrition* to begin re-designing your nutritional health immediately. Already a collector's item, *The Pro-Vita!* will soon go out of print. Its nutritional wisdom has already helped thousands experience the energy and joy of vitality that comes with living in the Optimal-Health Dimension. What you eat becomes the foundation of health or the cause of disease. Start now with *The Pro-Vita!* and build a new future of the best health.

Books

THE PRO-VITA! PLAN FOR OPTIMAL NUTRITION by Jack Tips

At last! A way to build health based on both biochemistry and bioenergy! An extraordinary overview of how to minimize stress and maximize assimilation of essential nutrients: ever-important vegetables, low-stress protein, essential oils, and carbohydrates. A safe, non-radical nutritional foundation for your healing program, abundant health, greater energy and longevity. Daily nutrition plans and delicious recipes are included. Learn how to design the optimal nutrition meal! A simple approach to more energy, weight loss, improved immunity, and better health. Truly a masterpiece of nutritional wisdom! 380 pages, index, ISBN 0-929167-05-8 ($19.95)

CONQUER CANDIDA – RESTORE YOUR IMMUNE SYSTEM by Jack Tips

An in-depth look at this health-undermining pandemic that contributes to allergies, chronic fatigue, PMS, chronic infections, headaches, bloating, memory loss, and immune deficiency; and explains what to do about it! Indicates causes and offers unique insights based on hundreds of clinical case histories. Information beyond current treatments offers understanding on how to conquer candida. Most informative book on subject to date. 163 pgs, ISBN 0-929167-00-7 ($14.95)

THE NEXT STEP TO GREATER ENERGY A unique perspective on bioenergy, addictions and transformation. by Jack Tips

Explore the energy systems of the body with emphasis on the glandular (thyroid and adrenals) and bio-electric energy systems. A new look at the connection between bioenergy and addictions, taking a new look at energy impostors including substances, activities, and habits. Identifies addictions and habits as symptoms of bioenergetic and biochemical imbalances. Helps to discover the true cause of cravings and addictive patterns, and how to correct the underlying imbalance. How to stop smoking is thoroughly discussed. The focus of this practical information is how to obtain freedom and fuller spiritual expression. When you are ready for change, you are ready for THE NEXT STEP! 210 pages, index, ISBN 0-929167-04-X ($15.95)

YOUR LIVER – YOUR LIFELINE! by Jack Tips

A fascinating look at the liver – your most important organ – its bioforces and the Chinese healing system involving the triad of the liver-stomach-colon. Explains in easy steps how to detoxify your liver and entire body the natural way. Contains provocative insights into how herbs work, natural liver treatment and cure. Featured at Anthony Robbins' *Life Mastery University.* 146 pgs, Illustrations, photos, index, ISBN 0-929167-06-6 ($12.95)

Manuals

THE ART & SCIENCE OF SCLEROLOGY CERTIFICATION COURSE by Jack Tips

The definitive work on the science of interpreting the red lines in the white of the eyes to understand how stresses are effecting the body. This manual documents the life work of

A.S. Wheelwright, preserving his great knowledge about this accurate and insightful health diagnostic tool. By studying this manual, you can become a master of understanding the hidden causes of health-stress manifesting in the body. A must for every iridologist and natural health care practitioner. Understand the language of the eyes and practice preventive health for yourself, your family, your friends. The course contains the 250-page, illustrated manual, seven hours of video tapes, acetate overlay charting system, wall chart, and certification exam. Regularly a $699 course, available by arrangement with the International Sclerology Institute at a discount. ISBN 0-929167-08-2 ($399.00)

Miscellaneous

WOMEN'S HEALTH DISCOURSES by Jack Tips

Four discourses: 1) PMS - Features a questionnaire for physical and emotional symptoms, and a guide to using emotional symptoms to design a complete nutritional program. Discusses the subject with insights few professionals consider. 2) A Systemic Approach to Menopause - The myths of menopause and how nutrition can help avoid the need for estrogen replacement. Provides programs for hot flashes, flooding, calcium utilization, insomnia and other post-menopausal conditions, 3) Osteoporosis: The Preventable Disease - A discussion of the causes and prevention of this disease, the osteoporosis equation, and an osteoporosis risk survey, and 4) Breast Health - The breast massage technique and its role in overall female endocrine health and the prevention of disease. Never published, manuscript form. 60 pages, 8 1/2 x 11", ($19.95)

Audio Offerings

THE HEALING TRIAD with Jack Tips

Master vibrant health in a polluted world! Learn about the healing triad, the truth about parasites, and a simple technique for detecting liver problems. Find out about the liver's role in allergies, PMS, candida, fatigue, and skin problems. In this lively discussion, you'll discover how to improve digestion, detoxification and elimination. 2 cassettes in binder ISBN 0-929167-13-9 ($19.95)

Ordering Information

A complete catalog is available on request featuring tapes, videos, courses and additional publications for health professionals.

Apple-A-Day Press
A Division of Apple-A-Day Enterprises, Inc.
3654 Bee Caves Road, Suite D
Austin, Texas 78746-5371

(512) 328-3996
FAX (512) 328-0812

e-mail: apple-a-day@jacktips.com
Order on the internet: www.jacktips.com

(Charges will include $3.95 shipping for one item plus $1.00 for each additional item.)

Mastercard, VISA, Discover, American Express, Checks

About The Author

by Robert Imbriale, President
Unlimited Leads, Inc., Chicago, IL

I first met Dr. Jack Tips in the summer of 1996 while attending Life Mastery University in Kona, Hawaii – a program hosted by world-renowned success coach, Anthony Robbins. At the time, what I did not know was that Dr. Tips was a renowned expert in nutrition, herbology, homeopathy, detoxification, and natural cure and that he was personally chosen by Tony Robbins to present his "groundbreaking" material to a standing ovation of more than 1,500 people. Tony introduced Jack as a "nutritional genius." I now know that was because of Jack's clear insights that can peer through the smokescreen of nutritional confusion and bring a common sense clarity to the seemingly complex issues that trouble the "experts."

Following his eye-opening presentation, I made my way through the crowd to meet him in person. I purchased a copy of his book, *"Your Liver – Your Lifeline."* About a year later, I contacted him again over the Internet to see if he had any new books available. A month later, during his travels, he and I had the opportunity to spend part of the afternoon together and it was then that I really got to know him.

Jack Tips is a man with a heart for people – all people. His life is dedicated to helping people lead healthy lives without the need for invasive procedures and harmful chemicals. But Dr. Tips has a much bigger mission in life. He is committed to finding a better way to feed the world's hungry populations with healthful, tasty, and affordable foods, as well as bring the message of health to the overfed but undernourished people subsisting on denatured foods.

Dr. Tips has studied with many of the world's most renowned natural health leaders, including: Dr. Herbert Shelton, Dr. Bernard Jensen, Stanley Burroughs, Dr. Paul Eck, Dr. Alan Beardall, Dr. Wilhelm Langreder, Dr. Francisco Eizayaga, Dr. Robin Murphy, and most notably as a protégé of Dr. A.S. Wheelwright, the master herbalist and sclerologist.

In the course of his many and varied studies, he earned an undergraduate degree from the University of Texas and a doctorate degree in Nutrition Science from the Roger Williams School of Nutrition Science. He is licensed as a Dietician/Nutritionist in New York. He is certified in classical homeopathy by the Hahnemann Academy of North America; in naturopathy by the American Naturopathic Medical Association; in clinical nutrition by the International and American Associations of Clinical Nutritionists.

His current natural health duties include:

- Director of the Apple-A-Day Clinic, Austin, TX
- CEO, International Sclerology Institute, Austin, TX
- Board of Directors, School of Natural Medicine, Santa Fe, NM
- Master Representative, Systemic Formulas, Ogden, UT
- Scientific Advisory Board for Ideal Health International, Boston, MA

Dr. Tips is so much more than an expert in natural health, he's a man with a passion for life and a vision of how to make life more enjoyable...naturally! I trust you have enjoyed this book and will take its advice to heart.